Topics in Postoperative Pain

Edited by Victor M. Whizar-Lugo,
Analucía Domínguez-Franco,
Marissa Minutti-Palacios
and Guillermo Dominguez-Cherit

Published in London, United Kingdom

Topics in Postoperative Pain
http://dx.doi.org/10.5772/intechopen.105661
Edited by Victor M. Whizar-Lugo, Analucía Domínguez-Franco, Marissa Minutti-Palacios and Guillermo Dominguez-Cherit

Contributors
Yetunde Oluwafunmilayo Tola, Ka Ming Chow, Wei Liang, Esther Ilesanmi, Oluwatosin Comfort Olarinde, Deborah Blessing Odejobi, K. Madan, Ramya B. Sriram, Lorena Bobadilla Suárez, Ailyn Cendejas Schotman, Jonathan Jair Mendoza Reyes, Luisa Fernanda Castillo Dávila, Fernando Mondragón Rodríguez, Navin Kumar, Rohik Anjum, Dhiraj Mallik, Farhanul Huda, Bibek Karki, Somprakas Basu, Pavla Pokorna, Hana Jancova, Ana Lilia Garduño-López, José Ramón Saucillo-Osuna, Eduardo Antonio Wilson-Manríquez, Mercedes Nicté López-Hernández, Ivet B. B. Koleva, Borislav R. Yoshinov, Teodora A. Asenova, Radoslav R. Yoshinov, Maiko Satomoto, Víctor M. Whizar-Lugo, Guillermo Domínguez-Cherit, Marissa Minutti-Palacios, Analucía Domínguez-Franco, Saúl Gilberto Almeida-Návar, Nexaí Reyes-Sampieri, Jose Trinidad Morelos-Garcia, Gabriel Ivan Herrejón-Galaviz, Jorge Mario Antolinez-Motta, Alejandro Escalona-Espinosa, Enrique Pazos-Alvarado, Kelly Maldonado-Sánchez, Rosina Alcaraz-Ramos, Pedro Castañeda, David Aguilar-Romero, Keisuke Lira-Hernandez, Lourdes Trinidad Castillo García, Fabiola Estela Elizabeth Ortega Ponce, Aurora Carolina Martínez Esparza, Daniela Arévalo-Villa, Andrea Figueroa Morales, Roberto de Jesús Jiménez-Contreras

First published in London, United Kingdom, 2023 by IntechOpen
IntechOpen is the global imprint of INTECHOPEN LIMITED, registered in England and Wales, registration number: 11086078, 5 Princes Gate Court, London, SW7 2QJ, United Kingdom

British Library Cataloguing-in-Publication Data
A catalogue record for this book is available from the British Library

Additional hard and PDF copies can be obtained from orders@intechopen.com

Topics in Postoperative Pain
Edited by Victor M. Whizar-Lugo, Analucía Domínguez-Franco, Marissa Minutti-Palacios and Guillermo Dominguez-Cherit
p. cm.
Print ISBN 978-1-83768-601-8
Online ISBN 978-1-83768-602-5
eBook (PDF) ISBN 978-1-83768-603-2

For EU product safety concerns:
IN TECH d.o.o., Prolaz Marije Krucifikse Kozulić 3, 51000 Rijeka, Croatia,
info@intechopen.com or visit our website at intechopen.com.

Meet the editors

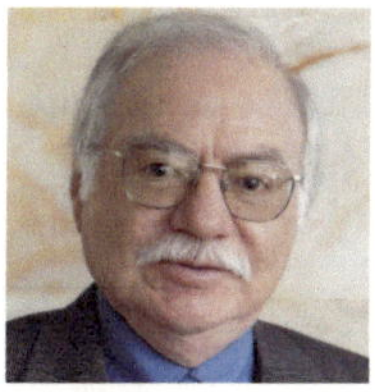

Víctor M. Whizar-Lugo, MD, graduated from Universidad Nacional Autónoma de México and completed his residency in internal medicine at Hospital General de México, Anesthesiology and Critical Care Medicine, Instituto Nacional de la Nutrición Salvador Zubirán, México City. He also completed a fellowship at the Anesthesia Department, Pain Clinic, University of California, Los Angeles, USA. Currently, Dr. Whizar-Lugo works in the Anesthesia Department at Lotus Med Group and is an associated researcher at the Institutos Nacionales de Salud, Mexico. He has publications on anesthesia, pain, internal medicine, and critical care to his credit. He has also edited five books and given countless conferences at congresses and meetings around the world. He is the editor-in-chief of the *Journal of Anesthesia* and *Critical Care*. Dr. Whizar-Lugo is the founding director of Anestesiología y Medicina del Dolor, a free medical education program on the Internet (www. anestesiologia-dolor. org).

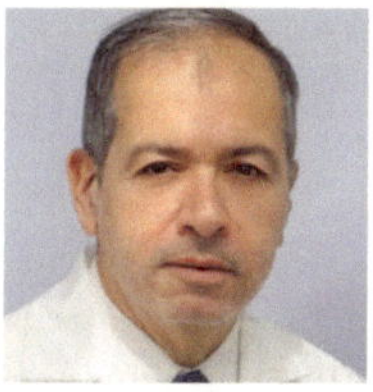

Guillermo Domínguez-Cherit, MD, graduated from the Faculty of Medicine, Universidad Nacional Autónoma de México and completed his residency in internal medicine, anesthesiology, and critical care medicine at Instituto Nacional de Ciencias Médicas y Nutrición Salvador Zubirán, México City. He also completed a professional internship in mechanical ventilation at Provincial Clinic Hospital I Barcelona and Sant Pau Barcelona Hospital, Spain. He is a member of the National Academy of Medicine of Mexico and of the Task Force of Mass Critical Care, American College of Chest Physicians. He is a researcher level II in the National System of Researchers in Mexico. Dr. Domínguez-Cherit is the deputy director of critical medicine at the Instituto Nacional de Ciencias Médicas y Nutrición Salvador Zubirán and the regional dean of the School of Medicine and Health Sciences, Monterrey Institute of Technology and Advanced Studies (ITESM), México City. He has been a visiting professor at national and international conferences and has published multiple investigations in journals and books.

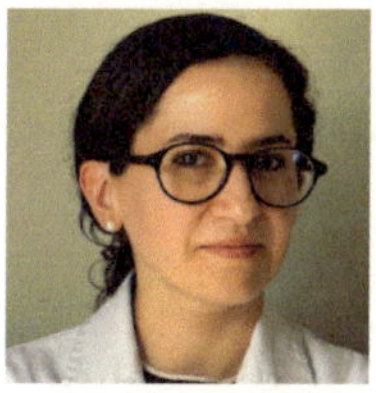

Marissa Minutti-Palacios, MD, graduated from the Faculty of Medicine, Universidad Popular Autónoma del Estado Puebla, México. She completed her residency in anesthesiology at the Instituto Nacional de Ciencias Médicas y Nutrición Salvador Zubirán, México City, and a fellowship in perioperative medicine of the obese patient at Centro Médico ABC, México City. She obtained a master's degree in Quantitative Methods for Health Research and Epidemiology at Universidad Autónoma de Madrid, Spain. Dr. Minutti-Palacios has publications in anesthesia and perioperative medicine to her credit and has lectured at conferences and meetings in México. She is a professor in the Faculty of Medicine, Tecnológico de Monterrey, México City.

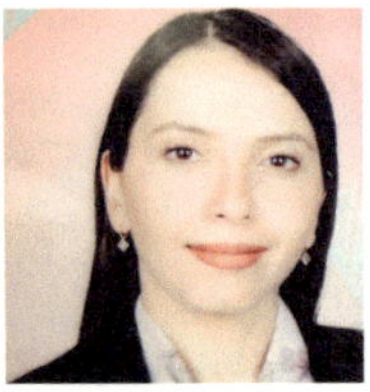

Analucía Domínguez-Franco, MD, graduated from the Faculty of Medicine, Universidad Anahuac Mayab, Yucatán, México. She completed her residency in anesthesiology and a fellowship in chronic pain and palliative medicine at the Instituto Nacional de Ciencias Médicas Y Nutrición Salvador Zubirán, México City. She has publications in chronic pain to her credit and has lectured at conferences and meetings in México. Currently, Dr. Domínguez-Franco is Professor of Anesthesiology in the Anesthesia Department, Instituto Nacional de Ciencias Médicas Y Nutrición Salvador Zubirán.

Contents

Preface

Postoperative pain (POP) is a health problem that has not yet been resolved. Without a doubt, multimodal analgesia is the greatest advance in the prevention and comprehensive management of patients with POP. Despite this advance, healthcare professionals require more knowledge to effectively manage POP since its deleterious effects manifest not only in the immediate post-surgical phase but can also be prolonged as postoperative chronic pain that is difficult to manage and interferes substantially with patient quality of life. In addition, poorly treated POP facilitates prolonged stays and/or hospital readmissions that increase care costs.

Opioids have long been the basis for the management of post-surgical pain. However, the overprescription of these drugs and their illegal use have led to the current opioid crisis worldwide, which has caused more than 96,700 deaths in the United States. The current trend is to reduce the use of opioids in pain management as well as search for new opioids with fewer side effects.

Topics in Postoperative Pain presents some selected subjects with the goal of improving the care of surgical patients and reducing both the sequelae of POP and the side effects of its management.

The editors of this book completed residencies at the same hospital, at very different times, with teachers and changing programs that have gradually adapted to the academic and care needs of our alma mater, the Instituto Nacional de Ciencias Médicas y Nutrición Salvador Zubirán. As graduates from the Division of Anesthesiology and Critical Care Medicine, we know about the goals, challenges, successes, and failures of the founders of our group and we wish to dedicate this book to them: Javier Ramírez Acosta, Ramon De Lille Fuentes, J. Antonio Jimenez Borreiro, and Gabriel Camacho Romero began training specialists in anesthesiology and critical medicine in 1972.

Thank you very much for your wisdom, your dedication, and above all your valuable friendship!

Victor M. Whizar-Lugo
Anesthesiologist,
Lotus Med Group,
Institutos Nacionales de Salud,
Tijuana, México

Guillermo Domínguez-Cherit
School of Medicine and Health Sciences,
School of Medicine,
Monterrey Institute of Technology and Advanced Studies (ITESM),
Ciudad de México, México

National Institute of Medical Sciences and Nutrition Salvador Zubirán,
Mexico City, Mexico

Marissa Minutti-Palacios
Faculty of Medicine,
Anesthesia Department,
Hospital ABC,
Monterrey Institute of Technology and Higher Education,
Ciudad de México, México

Analucía Domínguez-Franco
Anesthesia Department,
National Institute of Medical Sciences and Nutrition Salvador Zubirán,
Ciudad de México, México

Chapter 1

Introductory Chapter: Understanding Postoperative Pain

Victor M. Whizar-Lugo, Guillermo Domínguez-Cherit, Marissa Minutti-Palacios and Analucía Domínguez-Franco

1. Introduction

Postoperative pain (POP) is the result of the aggression of the surgical scalpel and sometimes of some anesthetic procedures. Both factors trigger a number of side effects including inflammation and nerve injury as a result of different pathophysiological mechanisms. This symptom can be devastating and does not have a useful biological function, which is why it is mandatory to prevent it, diagnose it, and treat it with a multimodal approach and thus reduce or avoid its multiple deleterious effects and, of course, reduce or evade the possibility of chronic postoperative pain (CPOP) [1, 2]. Despite advances in the comprehensive management of POP, its incidence could reach 86% of people who undergo surgery and suffer from moderate or severe POP on the first postoperative day [3]. Fortunately, physicians are now more interested in the proper management of POP and we have multiple resources to prevent and treat it more effectively and safely.

There are recognized factors for developing POP, such as age, pain prior to surgery, general anesthesia, long-term surgery, and some types of surgery, such as mastectomy, cesarean section, amputation, etc. [4].

Proper management of POP includes drugs, anesthesia techniques, enhanced recovery pathways in surgery and anesthesia, as well as non-pharmacological modalities. At present, multimodal analgesia combines all these management modalities and it has been shown that the postoperative evolution is better and with a clear decrease in the consumption of opioids [5], which is essential in this critical period of legal and illegal use of narcotic drugs.

The crisis of using illegal fentanyl mixed with other narcotics is a factor that should interest us in relation to a more rational management of opioids in the perioperative period. Although fentanyl and morphine have a prominent place in the management of POP, patients taking opioids prior to surgery have been found to be at high risk of continuing this habit even after they have recovered from their surgery.

The objective of this introductory chapter to our book on topics in postsurgical pain is the understanding of POP, its management, and repercussions on the evolution of patients.

IntechOpen

2. Anatomy and physiology

Surgical tissue trauma leads to nociceptive activation and sensitization. POP is caused by surgical incision, inflammation, and nerve injury as a result of different pathophysiological mechanisms. Acute POP is described as nociceptive pain that is well localized and characterized as sharp, aching, and throbbing, triggered by myelinated A-delta and slow conducting unmyelinated C-fiber nociceptors that are sensitized by an incision [6] and this is better known as nociceptive pain [7]. Nociceptive input from A-delta and C fibers enters the spinal cord via the dorsal horn and synapses with second-order neurons at A-delta at laminae II and V, and C and laminae II. From here, pain signals cross to ascending spinothalamic and spinoreticular pathways to ultimately reach higher brain centers. The spinothalamic tract is considered the main pain pathway and originates from the neurons in laminae I and V–VII. This tract synapses with third-order neurons in the thalamus. The spinoreticular pathway synapses in the brainstem with projections to the thalamus, hypothalamus, and cortex and this is the pathway that is involved in the emotional and psychological experience of pain [6].

Inflammatory responses are involved in acute POP. This response is induced by a surgical tissue injury that originates a cascade of events that result in an expression of mediators including prostaglandins, interleukins, cytokines, and neurotrophin-like nerve growth factor (NGF), glial-derived neurotrophic factor (GDNF), neurotrophin-3 (NT-3) and neurotrophin-5 (NT-5), and brain-derived neurotrophic factor (BDNF) [7, 8]. These mediators lead to a reduction in the threshold that innervates the injured tissues and explains peripheral sensitization [8–10]. The prostanoid production at the site of surgical injury results from the generation of arachidonic acid from membrane phospholipids by phospholipase A2. Cyclooxygenase-2 (COX-2) converts arachidonic acid into prostaglandin H, which is converted into specific prostanoid species, such as prostaglandin E2, by prostaglandin synthases. The prostanoid prostaglandin E2 and NGF bind to G-protein-coupled prostaglandin E and tyrosine kinase A receptors, respectively, to modify the sensitivity of the terminal without emitting direct nociceptor activation [10]. Central sensitization is a form of synaptic plasticity in the neurons from the dorsal horn of the spinal cord or in the spinal nucleus of the trigeminal nerve. This type of sensitization describes the phenomenon of amplifying pain signaling and it requires concise but intense nociceptor activity to be initiated, like a surgical incision. The repeated low-frequency activation of C fibers and the glutamate-activated N-methyl-D-aspartate (NMDA) receptor are closely involved in this sensitization pathway. The descending noradrenergic pathways are inhibitory and modulate nociceptive transmission and spinal sensitization. The rostroventromedial medulla (RVM) and adjacent areas though the dorsal horn of the spinal cord transmit in a descending way the pathways originated in the cortex and thalamus. These areas of the brainstem also receive afferent input from the superficial dorsal horn, periaqueductal gray (PAG), nucleus tractus solitarius (NTS), and parabrachial nucleus [11]. The descending and inhibitory pathways minimize the nociceptive transmission via noradrenaline, stimulating alpha 2 (a2)-adrenoceptors and serotonin [12].

3. Evaluating POP

The assessment of POP is of paramount importance in the comprehensive management of surgical patients. Pain intensity assessment should be done with a pain

• Visual analog scales (VAS)
• Verbal rating scale (VRS)
• Numerical rating scale (NRS)
• Faces pain scale (FPS)
• Heft-Parker visual analog scale (HPS)
• The Non-Communicating Children's Pain Checklist-Postoperative Version (NCCPC-PV)
• Face, Legs, Activity, Cry, Consolability (FLACC)
• Wong-Baker faces pain rating scale (WBS)

Table 1.
Scales to measure pain.

scale. POP is most often measured using unidimensional pain scales. While there are many different pain scales available, the visual analog scale (VAS) is the most commonly used scale. This scale involves the use of a metric line marked from 0 to 10 with verbal descriptions of pain at either end of the scale, with 0 representing "no pain" and 10 representing "worst possible pain." Since the original description of VAS [13], various measurement tools have been described and validated to assess acute and chronic pain as observed in **Table 1** [14–16]. In adults, the VAS, verbal rating scale (VRS), and numerical rating scale (NRS) are the most used due to their ease and veracity of the data obtained. When adult patients have some cognitive deficiency, it is prudent to use other scales such as those used with emoji faces as described by Li et al. [17] for patients to assess their pain on mobile devices and found that this form of assessment was reliable and valid compared with traditional pain scales in adult surgery patients. Analgesic management that delivers a change of 10 for the 100 mm pain VAS signifies a clinically important improvement or deterioration, and a VAS of 33 or less signifies satisfactory POP control [15].

In pediatrics, it is mandatory to assess pain with special scales designed for different ages; neonates, children, or adolescents [18–20]. In children with cognitive deficiency, the nonverbal expressions of pain should be used. The Non-Communicating Children's Pain Checklist-Postoperative Version (NCCPC-PV) and the Face, Legs, Activity, Cry, and Consolability (FLACC) scales have proven to be reliable [21].

4. Preventing acute postoperative pain

As we mentioned, inadequate pain management after surgery increases the risk of postoperative complications and may predispose for chronic postsurgical pain. The original idea of preventing pain is attributed to George W. Crile who in 1912 described what he called anoci-nociception; before starting the surgery, he injected parenteral morphine and local cocaine to block the transmission of painful stimulation [22–24]. Years later, Woolf [25, 26], Dickenson [27], and Wall [28] evidenced that administration of opioids or local anesthetics before noxious stimulus can prevent the development of injured-spinal hyperexcitability and pain-related behavior. The first clinical investigation on preemptive analgesia was published by Tverskoy in 1990 [29]. Since then, the prevention and management of POP has evolved based on these facts and its solid evolution is founded on advances in pharmacology and the various techniques of anesthesia, surgical and non-pharmacological approaches, as described

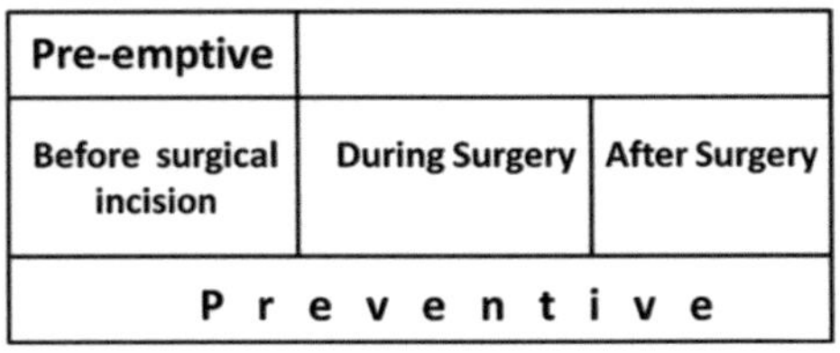

Figure 1.
Pre-emptive analgesia is accomplished with analgesics, local anesthetics and adjuvants drugs given before surgery begins. Preventive analgesia refers to drugs given before, during and after surgery [24].

in the chapters of this book. **Figure 1** shows Crile's original idea as it is used today. As seen in **Table 2**, there are several drugs that are used in the preemptive and preventive management of POP.

The side effects mentioned in **Table 2** are infrequent, sometimes dose-dependent, and should not be a limitation in the prescription of these drugs, except when there is any formal contraindication or history of adverse reactions, including known allergies [29–36].

Pre-emptive and preventive drugs	Pharmacological name	Side effects
Paracetamol	Acetaminophen	Agitation, constipation, headaches, insomnia, itchy gastritis, liver damage,
Dipyrone	Metamizole sodium	Hypotension, chest pain and arrhythmias, nausea, dizziness, kidney damage, shortness of breath, rash, severe allergy, Stevens-Johnson syndrome, Lyell's syndrome, hemolytic anemia, aplastic anemia, agranulocytosis, thrombocytopenia, pancytopenia.
Alfa2 agonists	Clonidine, Dexmedetomidine	Drowsiness, bradycardia, arterial hypotension, transient hypertension
Gabapentinoids	Gabapentin, pregabalin	Drowsiness, weakness or tiredness, dizziness, headache, tremor, double or blurred vision, Instability, anxiety, nausea and vomiting
Ketamine	S(+)-ketamine, (R)-ketamine	Dream-like feeling, blurred vision, double vision, jerky muscle movements, dizziness, drowsiness, nausea, vomiting, confusion, hallucinations, unusual thoughts, extreme fear.
Magnesium	Magnesium sulphate	• Confusion, dizziness or lightheadedness, irregular heartbeat, hypotension, sleepiness, muscle weakness
NSAIDs	Celecoxib, diclofenac, etoricoxib ibuprofen, ketorolac, meloxicam, naproxen, parecoxib	• Gastritis and gastric ulcers, indigestion, diarrhea, headaches, drowsiness, dizziness, allergic reactions.

Pre-emptive and preventive drugs	Pharmacological name	Side effects
Opioids	Morphine, fentanyl, methadone, buprenorphine, tramadol, codeine. Oliceridine	Respiratory depression, arterial hypotension, bradycardia, delirium, drug addiction
Steroids	dexamethasone	Hypertension, peptic ulcers, hyperglycemia, and hydro-electrolytic disorders.
Miscellaneous	Levitracepam, esmolol	

Table 2.
Most used analgesic and adjuvant pre-emptive and preventive drugs.

5. Postsurgical pain management

The prevention and management of POP requires a complete knowledge of the anatomy, physiology, and pharmacology of the elements involved: from molecular receptors to psychological aspects in such a way that we can structure a perioperative multimodal analgesic plan [5, 8, 9, 11, 34]. The American Society of Anesthesiologists (ASA) and other similar societies have published various guidelines for the multidisciplinary management of POP [37–39].

The timely identification of risk factors [1, 3, 4] for patients to develop severe or difficult-to-manage POP is of vital importance to plan a preemptive and preventive pain management. For example, prolonged surgeries with extensive tissue damage, potential for neural injury, multiple simultaneous operative sites, oncologic and orthopedic procedures, and breast surgery produce POP more frequently. In a study of 11,510 patients from 26 countries, it was found that POP decreases with increasing age, although this decrease in pain is of questionable clinical importance [3].

In this clinical setting, it is accepted that the combination of various therapeutic approaches—multimodal analgesia—is currently the most effective and safe treatment, reduces the consumption of opioids, as well as decreases postoperative nausea and vomiting [5]. **Table 3** mentions the most common management approaches.

Recently, some countries are experiencing a severe opioid consumption crisis in which the legal prescription and the unlawful use of these drugs are determining factors in the alarming increase in mortality related to the use of opioids, particularly fentanyl [40]. A multicenter study of 1093 major surgery cases found that the most important variable in opioid use 3 months after surgery was preoperative opioid use [41]. The current trend is to reduce opioids during and after surgery whenever possible with the goal of curbing opioid-related morbidity and mortality and engaging in the safe and rational management of POP [42]. Opioid-free anesthesia is a strong proposition in the midst of this global opioid consumption crisis [43–46]. However, the reduction of opioids in the perioperative period, especially in the management of POP, requires more aggressive programs among anesthesiologists, surgeons, and nurses.

There is a recent advance in the pharmacological management of POP; the new drug oliceridine is an innovative mu-opioid receptor agonist that is part of a new group of biased ligands that selectively activate G-protein signaling and downregulate

Pain medicines • Analgesics • Local anesthetics • Adjuvants
Local anesthetics / Regional anesthetic techniques Topical techniques • Local • anesthetic wound infiltration • Intra-articular • Intravenous blocks (IVRA) Neuroaxial • Spinal • Epidural Nerve blocks • Paravertebral blocks • Plexus nerve block • Peripheral nerve blocks • Fascial plane block • Interpleural analgesia
Patient-controlled analgesia (PCA)
Examples of non-pharmacologic therapies • Cognitive modalities • Physical therapy • Transcutaneous electrical nerve stimulation (TENS) • Acupuncture, massage • Music • Physical Heat, ice/cooling • Activities Hobbies/leisure • Hypnosis • Spiritual religious literature and services

Table 3.
Drugs, and procedures used in the comprehensive management of POP.

β-arrestin recruitment. Since G-protein signaling has been associated with analgesia while β-arrestin recruitment has been related to opioid adverse events, there is potential for a wider therapeutic window, including postoperative analgesia. It has been approved by the Food and Drug Administration (FDA) for the treatment of moderate-to-severe postoperative acute pain. Its analgesic efficacy has been found to be similar to that of morphine, with a profile of fewer side effects. More clinical studies are required to determine its role in the management of POP [47–50].

Obese and opioid use disorder patients are a challenge in opioid administration for POP. Regional anesthesia techniques and trying to avoid opioids are preferred analgesic approaches, with multimodal analgesia being the technique of choice.

Comprehensive management of POP should include the non-pharmacological approaches listed in **Table 3**. Some perioperative psychological techniques can decrease the intensity of POP and thereby reduce the use of opioids in POP [51].

6. Acute complications of POP

Inadequate postoperative analgesia induces adverse consequences in the immediate postoperative period and favors CPOP. Nowadays, literature suggests that severe acute

Complications	
Deep vein thrombosis and/or PE	**Postoperative cognitive dysfunction**
Pulmonary infections, respiratory depression	Prolonged hospitalization, unplanned hospital admissions
Myocardial ischemia and infarction	Increase in the price of care
Paralytic ileus, urinary retention	Rebound pain / Chronic postoperative pain
Complications related to analgesia modalities: Somnolence, sedation, dizziness, respiratory depression, urinary retention, nausea/vomiting, ileus, pruritus, risk of addiction/substance use disorder, gastrointestinal bleeding, renal dysfunction, transient motor blockade, etc	Disability to perform activities of daily living, impaired ability to sleep, low mood, and decreased libido

Table 4.
Complications related to inadequate POP management.

POP is common, though most of the time it is underestimated and often inadequately treated (**Table 4**). Ineffective postoperative acute pain control is associated with poor outcomes including increased length-of-stay, sleep disturbance, prolonged time to first mobilization, and increased opioid use. Furthermore, poor postoperative pain control has been associated with delirium in the elderly, cardiopulmonary and thromboembolic complications [52]. POP not only affects patient health, but it may also increase the risk of developing chronic pain and its consequences. Fletcher et al. [53] reported that every 10% increase in the time spent in severe postoperative pain was associated with a 30% increase in chronic pain 12 months after surgery. Tissue injury generates an allostatic response that involves nervous, endocrine, and immune processes. Initially, the physiologic response to acute pain is adaptive, as it facilitates an immediate response via the sympathetic nervous system and the neuroendocrine system [54]. As the autonomic nervous system may be activated during an acute painful event, different changes in vital signs like the elevation of systolic blood pressure (SBP), diastolic blood pressure (DBP), mean arterial pressure (MAP), and pulse rate (PR) are recorded. These changes could be suggestive of the presence of discomfort or pain like how some studies show in the intensive care unit (ICU) population [55]. Willingham et al. [56] analyzed a cohort that included 11,986 adult postsurgical patients, and the most common type of postoperative complication was wound infection (3.6%), followed by respiratory (3.0%), neural (2.8%), cardiac (2.5%), thrombotic (2.5%), and renal/gastrointestinal (2.0%). Patients with severe pain experienced an overall complication rate of 15.9% versus that of 12.4% in those patients without. Its key factor not only focuses on controlling PAP, but is also necessary to systematically identify significant preoperative predictors of poorly controlled acute postoperative pain and to quantify the associated risks. It has been hypothesized that adequate pain control represents a reduction in the surgical stress responses (endocrine, metabolic, and inflammatory), therefore improving analgesia will lead to a reduced incidence of postoperative organ dysfunction and result in a better outcome.

7. Conclusions

Management of acute postoperative pain is a major challenge for clinicians, with more than 80% of patients reporting pain after surgery and 75% reporting pain that is moderate, severe, or even extreme, although these figures vary according to factors, such as the age and sex of the patient, certain preoperative factors, biopsychosocial factors, the type and duration of surgery, the analgesic/anesthetic intervention used, and the time elapsed after surgery. This may favor CPOP. It is vitally important to identify the risk factors for POP and establish perioperative management plans using the techniques described, multimodal analgesia being the most effective procedure. Emphasizing a multimodal analgesic approach and an individualized plan for the management of POP significantly reduces the demand for opioids while optimizing pain relief and speedy recovery of patients.

Author details

Victor M. Whizar-Lugo[1*], Guillermo Domínguez-Cherit[2,3], Marissa Minutti-Palacios[4] and Analucía Domínguez-Franco[5]

1 Anesthesiologist at Lotus Med Group, Institutos Nacionales de Salud, Tijuana, México

2 School of Medicine and Health Sciences, School of Medicine, Monterrey Institute of Technology and Advanced Studies (ITESM), Ciudad de México, México

3 National Institute of Medical Sciences and Nutrition Salvador Zubirán, Mexico City, Mexico

4 Faculty of Medicine, Anesthesia Department, Hospital ABC, Tecnológico de Monterrey, Ciudad de México, México

5 Anesthesia Department, Instituto Nacional de Ciencias Médicas y Nutrición Salvador Zubirán, Ciudad de México, México

*Address all correspondence to: vwhizar@anestesia-dolor.org and vwhizarl@gmail.com

References

[1] Coppes OJM, Yong RJ, Kaye AD, Urman RD. Patient and surgery-related predictors of acute postoperative pain. Current Pain and Headache Reports. 2020;**24**(4):12. DOI: 10.1007/s11916-020-0844-3

[2] O'Neill A, Lirk P. Multimodal Analgesia. Anesthesiology Clinics. 2022;**40**(3):455-468. DOI: 10.1016/j.anclin.2022.04.002

[3] van Dijk JFM, Zaslansky R, van Boekel RLM, Cheuk-Alam JM, Baart SJ, Huygen FJPM, et al. Postoperative pain and age: A retrospective cohort association study. Anesthesiology. 2021;**135**(6):1104-1119. DOI: 10.1097/ALN.0000000000004000

[4] Wang Y, Liu Z, Chen S, Ye X, Xie W, Hu C, et al. Pre-surgery beliefs about pain and surgery as predictors of acute and chronic post-surgical pain: A prospective cohort study. International Journal of Surgery. 2018;**52**:50-55. DOI: 10.1016/j.ijsu.2018.02.032

[5] Hinther A, Nakoneshny SC, Chandarana SP, Matthews TW, Hart R, Schrag C, et al. Efficacy of multimodal analgesia for postoperative pain management in head and neck cancer patients. Cancers (Basel). 2021;**13**(6):1266. DOI: 10.3390/cancers13061266

[6] Xuan C, Yan W, Wang D, Li C, Ma H, Mueller A, et al. Efficacy of preemptive analgesia treatments for the management of postoperative pain: A network meta-analysis. British Journal of Anaesthesia. 2022;**129**(6):946-958. DOI: 10.1016/j.bja.2022.08.038

[7] Mazda Y, Jadin S, Khan JS. Postoperative pain management. Canadian Journal of General Internal Medicine. 2021;**16**:5-15. DOI: 10.22374/cjgim.v16iSP1.529

[8] Henrik K, Jensen Troels S, Woolf CJ. Persistent postsurgical pain: Risk factors and prevention. Lancet. 2006;**367**:1618-1625

[9] Carvalho B, Clark DJ, Angst MS. Local and systemic release of cytokines, nerve growth factor, prostaglandin E2, and substance P in incisional wounds and serum following cesarean delivery. Journal of Pain. 2008;**9**(7):650-657

[10] Margraf A, Ludwig N, Zarbock A, Rossaint J. Systemic inflammatory response syndrome after surgery: Mechanisms and protection. Anesthesia and Analgesia. 2020;**131**(6):1693-1707. DOI: 10.1213/ANE.0000000000005175

[11] Vane JR, Bakhle YS, Botting RM. Cyclooxygenases 1 and 2. Annual Review of Pharmacology and Toxicology. 1998;**38**:97-120. DOI: 10.1146/annurev.pharmtox.38.1.97

[12] Heinricher MM, Tavares I, Leith JL, Lumb BM. Descending control of nociception: Specificity, recruitment and plasticity. Brain Research Reviews. 2009;**60**:214-225

[13] Feizerfan A, Sheh G. Transition from acute to chronic pain. Continuing Education in Anaesthesia Critical Care & Pain. 2015;**15**(2):98-102. DOI: 10.1093/bjaceaccp/mku044

[14] Hayes MHS, Patterson DG. Experimental development of the graphic rating method. Psychological Bulletin. 1921;**18**:98-99

[15] Karcioglu O, Topacoglu H, Dikme O, Dikme O. A systematic review of the pain scales in adults: Which to use? The American Journal of Emergency Medicine. 2018;**36**(4):707-714. DOI: 10.1016/j.ajem.2018.01.008

[16] Myles PS, Myles DB, Galagher W, Boyd D, Chew C, MacDonald N, et al. Measuring acute postoperative pain using the visual analog scale: The minimal clinically important difference and patient acceptable symptom state. British Journal of Anaesthesia. 2017;**118**(3):424-429. DOI: 10.1093/bja/aew466

[17] Li L, Wu S, Wang J, Wang C, Zuo W, Yu L, et al. Development of the emoji faces pain scale and its validation on mobile devices in adult surgery patients: Longitudinal observational study. Journal of Medical Internet Research. 2023;**25**:e41189. DOI: 10.2196/41189

[18] Kamki H, Kalaskar RR, Balasubramanian S. Evaluation of effectiveness of graphics interchange format and Wong-baker FACES pain rating scale as pain assessment tool in children. The Journal of Contemporary Dental Practice. 2022;**23**(6):634-638

[19] Maxwell LG, Fraga MV, Malavolta CP. Assessment of pain in the newborn: An update. Clinics in Perinatology. 2019;**46**(4):693-707. DOI: 10.1016/j.clp.2019.08.005

[20] Zieliński J, Morawska-Kochman M, Zatoński T. Pain assessment and management in children in the postoperative period: A review of the most commonly used postoperative pain assessment tools, new diagnostic methods and the latest guidelines for postoperative pain therapy in children. Advances in Clinical and Experimental Medicine. 2020;**29**(3):365-374. DOI: 10.17219/acem/112600

[21] Pizzinato A, Liguoro I, Pusiol A, Cogo P, Palese A, Vidal E. Detection and assessment of postoperative pain in children with cognitive impairment: A systematic literature review and meta-analysis. European Journal of Pain. 2022;**26**(5):965-979. DOI: 10.1002/ejp.1936

[22] Crile GW, Lower WE. Anoci-Association. In: Rowland AF, editor. First ed. Philadelphia and London: WB Saunders Company; 1914

[23] Katz J. George Washington Crile, anoci-association, and pre-emptive analgesia. Pain. 1993;**53**:243-245

[24] Whizar-Lugo VM. One century of pre-emptive and preventive analgesia. A tribute to George Washington Crile. Journal of Anesthesia and Critical Care: Open Access. 2014, 2014;**1**(5):00032. DOI: 10.15406/jaccoa.2014.01.00032

[25] Woolf CJ. Evidence for a central component of post-injury pain hypersensitivity. Nature. 1983;**306**(5944):686-688

[26] Woolf CJ, Chong MS. Preemptive analgesia-treating postoperative pain by preventing the establishment of central sensitization. Anesthesia and Analgesia. 1993;**77**:362-379

[27] Dickenson AH, Sullivan AF. Subcutaneous formalin-induced activity of dorsal horn neurones in the rat: Differential response to an intrathecal opiate administered pre or post formalin. Pain. 1987;**30**(3):349-360. DOI: 10.1016/0304-3959(87)90023-6

[28] Wall PD. The prevention of postoperative pain. Pain. 1988;**33**:289-290

[29] Tverskoy M, Cozacov C, Ayache M, Bradley EL, Kissin I. Postoperative

pain after inguinal herniorraphy with different types of anesthesia. Anesthesia and Analgesia. 1990;**70**:29-35

[30] Brinck EC, Tiippana E, Heesen M, Bell RF, Straube S, Moore RA, et al. Perioperative intravenous ketamine for acute postoperative pain in adults. Cochrane Database of Systematic Reviews. 2018;**12**(12):CD012033. DOI: 10.1002/14651858.CD012033.pub4

[31] Schwenk ES, Viscusi ER, Buvanendran A, Hurley RW, Wasan AD, Narouze S, et al. Consensus guidelines on the use of intravenous ketamine infusions for acute pain management from the American Society of Regional Anesthesia and Pain Medicine, the American Academy of pain medicine, and the American Society of Anesthesiologists. Regional Anesthesia and Pain Medicine. 2018;**43**(5):456-466. DOI: 10.1097/AAP.0000000000000806

[32] Wang H, Duan C, Zhang J, Qu S, Sun Y, Zhou L, et al. Evaluation of the effect of perioperative administration of S(+)-ketamine hydrochloride injection for postoperative acute pain in children: Study protocol for a prospective, multicenter, randomized, open-label, parallel-group, pragmatic clinical trial. Trials. 2022;**23**(1):586. DOI: 10.1186/s13063-022-06534-z

[33] Khalil BNM, Elderh MSH, Khaja MAR, El-Shaer AN, Ali BEEH, Taeimah MOA. Perioperative use of ketamine infusion versus dexmedetomidine infusion for analgesia in obese patients undergoing bariatric surgery: A double-blinded three-armed randomized controlled trial. BMC Anesthesiology. 2023;**23**(1):108. DOI: 10.1186/s12871-023-02059-3

[34] Tubog TD. Overview of multimodal analgesia initiated in the perioperative setting. Journal of Perioperative Practice. 2021;**31**(5):191-198. DOI: 10.1177/1750458920928843

[35] Silva Filho SE, Sandes CS, Vieira JE, Cavalcanti IL. Analgesic effect of magnesium sulfate during total intravenous anesthesia: Randomized clinical study. Brazilian Journal of Anesthesiology. 2021;**71**(5):550-557. DOI: 10.1016/j.bjane.2021.02.008

[36] Whizar-Lugo VM, Granados M, De Lille FR, Gómez-Gutiérrez C, Zepeda-Mendoza AD. Alternativas de analgesia: interacciones entre fármacos y receptores. Actas Peruanas de Anestesiol. 2013;**21**:26-42

[37] American Society of Anesthesiologists Task Force on Acute Pain Management. Practice guidelines for acute pain management in the perioperative setting: An updated report by the American Society of Anesthesiologists Task Force on acute pain management. Anesthesiology. 2012;**116**(2):248-273. DOI: 10.1097/ALN.0b013e31823c1030

[38] Chou R, Gordon DB, de Leon-Casasola OA, Rosenberg JM, Bickler S, et al. Management of postoperative pain: A clinical practice guideline from the American pain society, the American Society of Regional Anesthesia and Pain Medicine, and the American Society of Anesthesiologists' committee on regional anesthesia, executive committee, and administrative council. The Journal of Pain. 2016;**17**(2):131-157. DOI: 10.1016/j.jpain.2015.12.008

[39] Small C, Laycock H. Acute postoperative pain management. The British Journal of Surgery. 2020;**107**(2):e70-e80. DOI: 10.1002/bjs.11477

[40] Upp LA, Waljee JF. The opioid epidemic. Clinics in Plastic Surgery.

2020;**47**(2):181-190. DOI: 10.1016/j.cps.2019.12.005

[41] Kuck K, Naik BI, Domino KB, Posner KL, Saager L, et al. Prolonged opioid use and pain outcome and associated factors after surgery under general anesthesia: A prospective cohort association multicenter study. Anesthesiology. 2023;**138**(5):462-476. DOI: 10.1097/ALN.0000000000004510

[42] Gabriel RA, Swisher MW, Sztain JF, Furnish TJ, Ilfeld BM, Said ET. State of the art opioid-sparing strategies for post-operative pain in adult surgical patients. Expert Opinion on Pharmacotherapy. 2019;**20**(8):949-961. DOI: 10.1080/14656566.2019.1583743

[43] Nicholas TA 4th, Robinson R. Multimodal analgesia in the era of the opioid epidemic. The Surgical Clinics of North America. 2022;**102**(1):105-115. DOI: 10.1016/j.suc.2021.09.003

[44] Rolfzen ML, Wick A, Mascha EJ, Shah K, Krause M, et al. Best practice alerts informed by inpatient opioid intake to reduce opioid prescribing after surgery (PRIOR) - a cluster randomized multiple crossover trial. Anesthesiology 2023;**138**. DOI: 10.1097/ALN.0000000000004607

[45] Beloeil H. Opioid-free anesthesia. Best Practice & Research. Clinical Anaesthesiology. 2019;**33**(3):353-360. DOI: 10.1016/j.bpa.2019.09.002

[46] Salomé A, Harkouk H, Fletcher D, Martinez V. Opioid-free anesthesia benefit-risk balance: A systematic review and meta-analysis of randomized controlled trials. Journal of Clinical Medicine. 2021;**10**(10):2069. DOI: 10.3390/jcm10102069

[47] Ayad S, Demitrack MA, Burt DA, Michalsky C, Wase L, et al. Evaluating the incidence of opioid-induced respiratory depression associated with oliceridine and morphine as measured by the frequency and average cumulative duration of dosing interruption in patients treated for acute postoperative pain. Clinical Drug Investigation. 2020;**40**(8):755-764. DOI: 10.1007/s40261-020-00936-0

[48] Daksla N, Wang A, Jin Z, Gupta A, Bergese SD. Oliceridine for the management of moderate to severe acute postoperative pain: A narrative review. Drug Design, Development and Therapy. 2023;**17**:875-886. DOI: 10.2147/DDDT.S372612

[49] Tan HS, Habib AS. Oliceridine: A novel drug for the management of moderate to severe acute pain - a review of current evidence. Journal of Pain Research. 2021;**14**:969-979. DOI: 10.2147/JPR.S278279

[50] Goudra B. Oliceridine-opioid of the 21st century. Saudi Journal of Anaesthesia. 2022;**16**(1):69-75. DOI: 10.4103/sja.sja_510_21

[51] Gorsky K, Black ND, Niazi A, Saripella A, Englesakis M, Leroux T, et al. Psychological interventions to reduce postoperative pain and opioid consumption: A narrative review of literature. Regional Anesthesia and Pain Medicine. 2021;**46**(10):893-903. DOI: 10.1136/rapm-2020-102434

[52] Yang MMH, Hartley RL, Leung AA, et al. Preoperative predictors of poor acute postoperative pain control: A systematic review and meta-analysis. BMJ Open. 2019;**9**:e025091

[53] Fletcher D, Stamer UM, Pogatzki-Zahn E, Zaslansky R, et al. Chronic postsurgical pain in Europe: An observational study. European Journal of

Anaesthesiology. 2015;**32**(10):725-734. DOI: 10.1097/EJA.0000000000000319

[54] Chapman CR, Tuckett RP, Song CW. Pain and stress in a systems perspective: Reciprocal neural, endocrine, and immune interactions. The Journal of Pain. 2008;**9**(2):122-145. DOI: 10.1016/j.jpain.2007.09.006

[55] Puntillo KA, Miaskowski C, Kehrle K, Stannard D, Gleeson S, Nye P. Relationship between behavioral and physiological indicators of pain, critical care patients' self-reports of pain, and opioid administration. Critical Care Medicine. 1997;**25**(7):1159-1166. DOI: 10.1097/00003246-199707000-00017.6

[56] Willingham M, Rangrass G, Curcuru C, Ben Abdallah A, Wildes TS, et al. Association between postoperative complications and lingering post-surgical pain: An observational cohort study. British Journal of Anaesthesia. 2020;**124**(2):214-221. DOI: 10.1016/j.bja.2019.10.012

Chapter 2

Changes in Postoperative Analgesia

Maiko Satomoto

Abstract

Postoperative pain management has changed with the evolution of surgical techniques. Epidural anesthesia was a very useful method of postoperative analgesia when laparotomy or thoracotomy was performed by making a large skin incision in the abdomen or chest. Nowadays, surgeries are often performed through very small skin incisions using laparoscopy or thoracoscopy. Furthermore, surgeries are often performed on elderly patients, and in many patients, anticoagulants are used in preoperative period and continued during intraoperative period or started early in postoperative period, and there are concerns that epidural anesthesia cannot be performed, or that epidural anesthesia may delay the start of early postoperative anticoagulation in such patients; hence, there is a tendency to avoid epidural anesthesia. In such cases, intravenous administration of patient-controlled analgesia (PCA) fentanyl is an effective method of postoperative analgesia. We will discuss the advantages and disadvantages of intravenous (IV)PCA and epidural anesthesia and also the combined use of peripheral nerve blocks, which has been in the spotlight in recent years. Early postoperative mobilization is useful in preventing muscle weakness and delirium. What we require today are postoperative analgesics that provide rapid postoperative recovery and do not cause nausea and vomiting.

Keywords: postoperative analgesia, surgery, laparoscopic surgery, IVPCA, epidural

1. Introduction

Postoperative pain is more than just the feeling of pain in the wound and is associated with damage to the tissues and organs involved in the surgical invasion. Postoperative pain consists of nociceptive pain, inflammatory pain, and neuropathic pain. In addition, psychogenic pain can also contribute to postoperative pain. Surgeries involving deep pain in bones, joints, or the spine and surgeries involving visceral pain, such as laparotomy, cause more severe postoperative pain than craniotomies or surgeries of the chest wall, abdominal wall, or skin, which cause only superficial pain. Postoperative pain is most severe during the first 24 hours following the surgery and often subsides thereafter, but in some cases, the pain may persist. In recent years, endoscopic surgeries with small skin incision account for the majority of planned surgeries. Although injuries to the skin and fascia have reduced, visceral injuries remain the same, which is why analgesics are necessary. In this section, we will discuss the changing approach to postoperative pain with the evolution of surgery and anesthesia.

2. Points to be noted before starting postoperative pain management

During the twentieth century, people came to increasingly believe that preoperative intervention was important when postoperative phase was taken into consideration. Perioperative management is a field that gives thought to what should be done to get patients into the best possible condition so that they can have a better postoperative comfort, by considering the preoperative, intraoperative, and postoperative phases seamlessly. Previously, anesthesiologists used to focus on intraoperative anesthesia management, but postoperative analgesic intervention, such as acute pain service (APS), has now developed with a focus on the management of postoperative pain as an extension of anesthesia, including epidural anesthesia. Postoperative wound pain is a problem common to all clinical departments, and it was 35 years ago that APS was proposed for pain management across departments [1]. Although many facilities have tried to standardize postoperative analgesia, there has been much debate about the service fee (cost calculation) of APS and the quality of analgesia, and questions were raised about the clinical utility of APS teams [2].

Meanwhile, there are known cases in which acute postoperative pain developed into chronic postoperative pain (CPSP). CPSP is defined as pain that persists for at least 3 months after surgery. Epidemiological studies report that CPSP occurs in 10–50% of patients undergoing surgery, and 2–10% have severe pain that interferes with daily life [3]. CPSP develops by a complex mechanism that includes surgical factors such as the extent of invasion, patient-related factors such as psychiatric and psychological factors and genetic predisposition, and environmental factors, and although knowing the exact pathology of CPSP is not simple, surgical technique, surgical wound size, duration of surgery, re-operation, and severe pain on the day following the surgery are also considered to be the causes of CPSP [4, 5]. It is important to note that CPSP that occurs as a result of inadequate management of this acute pain associated with surgery is considered as a problem, and the quality of postoperative analgesia is a major concern for patients when being referred to a hospital [6]. In the traditional postoperative management, the surgeon was the primary caregiver, who gave instructions to the nurse when the patient felt pain, and it often took about an hour from the time the patient complained of pain until the nurse comprehended the fact and administered analgesics to the patient.

3. Guidelines on postoperative pain

The American Pain Society, the American Society of Regional Anesthesia, and the American Society of Anesthesiologists jointly published Clinical Practice Guidelines on Postoperative Pain in 2016 [7]. The guidelines contain 32 recommendations, ranging from education of clinical staff and patients to specific surgical techniques. It is of concern that the level of evidence is not uniform, and that the contents of the recommendations vary widely. The important point is that if one wants to provide postoperative analgesia properly, then an environment should be provided in which the level of postoperative analgesia and its side effects can be objectively assessed for each surgery, starting with education in the preoperative outpatient setting, and the treatment plan for postoperative analgesia can be modified accordingly. It has been stated in the guidelines that it is efficient to collect medical information, formulate a plan for analgesia based on this information, and provide medical care by taking advantage of the specialties of the staff. In particular, with regard to analgesics to be used in the perioperative period, the guidelines discuss the importance of assessing the patient in the preoperative outpatient setting, formulating a plan for postoperative analgesia, and fully explaining the plan to the family and patient. The method of using the patient-controlled analgesia (PCA) pump and so on is hard to understand for the patient in an outpatient setting with an explanation from the anesthesiologist alone, and it is useful if the scrub nurse repeats the explanation. It is important to openly tell the ward nurse if one feels postoperative pain, and some facilities also need a change of mindset of the entire hospital from tolerating postoperative pain to finding remedies for it within the hospital. Reducing patient pain, reducing CPSP, and improving the reputation of the hospital go hand in hand, for which the collaboration between ward staff and operating room is important. It is also recommended that a scale be used to quantify pain. It is important to share information based on a uniform scale within the hospital and not based on subjectivity. Currently, Visual Analog Scale (VAS), Verbal Rating Scale (VRS), and Numerical Rating Scale (NRS) are available for the evaluation of pain. Postoperative analgesia is a basic requirement of perioperative care, and it is desirable to protocolize the evaluation and management of postoperative analgesia. There are cases in which observation of the patient's general condition is necessary in conjunction with analgesia, and this applies to cases in which spinal or epidural anesthesia is used, and although it is stated that multidisciplinary collaboration is necessary to provide an environment for monitoring [7], specific suggestions are not included in these guidelines. In Europe, a group of anesthesiologists and surgeons called Prospect (procedure specific postoperative pain management), led by the European Society of Regional Anesthesia, has proposed evidence-based analgesia for postoperative pain for each procedure [8–10]. In this proposal, optimal analgesics and regional anesthesia techniques are described in detail for each procedure.

4. Differences between laparotomy and laparoscopy

Since laparotomy is invasive and causes severe postoperative pain, postoperative analgesia plays an important role in early mobilization and shortening of hospital stay. Recently, there have been many cases of high-risk patients with venous thrombosis, atrial fibrillation, ischemic heart disease, and hemodialysis, who are being administered antiplatelet and anticoagulant drugs just before the surgery, and an epidural anesthesia cannot be used in many such patients. In these cases, intravenous patient-controlled analgesia (IV-PCA) is combined with peripheral nerve blocks of the abdominal wall.

On the other hand, laparoscopic surgery has advantages over laparotomy, such as smaller surgical incision, quicker postoperative recovery, and shorter hospital stay, and in recent years, almost all thoracic and abdominal surgeries tend to be performed by thoracoscopy or laparoscopy. While the monitor screen used during laparoscopy allows the medical staff to monitor the progress of the surgery, the field of view is limited, and it is necessary to be aware of unexpected bleeding or organ damage. There are advantages such as less postoperative pain compared to laparotomy and reduction in perioperative complications, including respiratory complications, due to early mobilization. The ability to tolerate the cardiorespiratory changes caused by insufflation and the cardiopulmonary effects due to body position must be evaluated prior to commencing the surgery. Epidural anesthesia is used in combination in cases where there is a high probability of conversion to laparotomy; otherwise, local infiltration anesthesia of the incision site is recommended in addition to intravenous patient-controlled analgesia (IV-PCA). Peripheral nerve blocks of the abdominal wall are also sometimes used in combination and are described for each laparoscopic procedure. For example, it is stated that in laparoscopic/robotic radical prostatectomy, bilateral transversus abdominis plane (TAP) block is recommended at the end of the procedure to reduce postoperative pain [11], while in laparoscopic cholecystectomy [10] and laparoscopic hysterectomy [12], TAP is recommended only when routine analgesia cannot be used for some reason, such as allergy. As there is no reliable large-scale research, the usefulness of peripheral nerve blocks has not been confirmed in the guidelines. In addition, laparoscopic surgery has a high incidence of postoperative nausea and vomiting; hence, preventive measures are necessary.

5. Problems specific to the elderly

Laparoscopy and thoracoscopy are becoming popular as surgical techniques because of their advantages such as they are less likely to cause postoperative leukocytosis, elevated c-reactive protein (CRP), and elevated blood glucose levels, resulting in shorter postoperative fasting time and hospital stay. As the population is aging, the elderly, who had avoided surgery in the past, are now proactively undergoing surgery with the popularization of the techniques that allow for rapid postoperative recovery. In Japan, 28.8% of the population is 65 years of age or older [12], and it is predicted that 2035 will see the onset of the aging society where one in three people will be 65 years of age or older. Even seemingly healthy elderly people have reduced vital functions and physiological reserves, and once complications occur, it takes time for them to recover.

Many patients who undergo surgical treatment have some comorbidity in the preoperative state. Complications such as diabetes, hypertension, chronic heart disease, chronic obstructive pulmonary disease, and chronic kidney disease and history of stroke are frequent and often concomitant. In planned surgeries, it is important to control remediable complications before surgery by performing additional examinations, where a multilateral, multidisciplinary approach to perioperative outpatient care becomes important. Patient care should include not only surgeons and anesthesiologists but also nurses, dental hygienists, rehabilitation specialists, and pharmacists, and the information shared before surgery should be passed on during intraoperative, postoperative, and recovery period. For multilateral preoperative risk assessment, anesthesiologists generally use the classification of preoperative physical status (PS) by the American Society of Anesthesiologists (ASA). MET, a unit measuring the intensity of a physical activity, indicates the intensity of an activity by how many times more energy is expended than when sitting quietly, which has a MET value of 1. How many METs of physical activity the patient is capable of is evaluated by quantifying the intensity of physical activities that the patient can perform daily. Generally, surgery is considered possible for patients with 4 MET.

6. Basal postoperative analgesics

Unless there are contraindications, acetaminophen and non-steroidal anti-inflammatory drugs (NSAIDs) are used as basal analgesics on a regular, rather than on an as-needed, basis for postoperative pain management. Treatment is switched to oral administration as soon as the patient is able to take drugs orally. Some Western protocols call for oral administration of acetaminophen, gabapentin, and celecoxib [6, 7, 9–11] 2 hours before surgery, but preoperative administration is not common in Japan. Similarly, postoperative gabapentin, though beneficial according to papers, is less common in Japan. This may be due to a lack of awareness about CPSP.

7. Benefits of epidural anesthesia

Epidural anesthesia is the administration of local anesthetics and sometimes opioids into the epidural space to provide analgesia. Epidural anesthesia may be used alone or in combination with spinal or general anesthesia. In addition to intraoperative analgesia, it is also used for postoperative analgesia with an indwelling catheter. Although this method of anesthesia provides good analgesia and is effective in facilitating mobilization, early detection of complications due to anesthesia is important.

Local anesthetics and opioids are used for epidural anesthesia. In recent years, opioids have been often avoided because of the serious complications that can occur in the case of inadvertent subarachnoid administration. The use of high concentrations of local anesthetics numbs not only the thin sensory nerves but also the thick motor nerves. Considering postoperative falls and delayed mobilization, there is a tendency to use low concentrations of local anesthetics. Local anesthesia alone is insufficient to cover movement pain, and using local anesthesia in combination with other analgesics to provide satisfactory postoperative analgesia is the current mainstream. Epidural anesthesia is superior in that it works in a segmental manner, allowing deep breathing and expectoration, with lesser postoperative respiratory complications, and in that the sympathetic nerve block allows rapid functional recovery of the gastrointestinal tract.

Compared to spinal anesthesia, its effect is milder, and the effect on circulation is also gradual. The main side effects are hypotension, bradycardia, and local anesthetic toxicity. The epidural space lies outside the dura mater and runs the entire length of the spinal canal. It extends from foramen magnum at its center to the sacrococcygeal ligament, covering the sacral hiatus at the caudal end, and laterally to the ligamentum flavum. Theoretically, epidural anesthesia can be used for any surgery except craniofacial surgeries, but it is often used for postoperative pain in thoracic and abdominal surgeries. Epidural anesthesia is also indicated for surgery of the lower extremities, but in recent years, there has been a tendency to perform peripheral nerve blocks since epidural anesthesia has an effect on both sides of the body.

Contraindications to epidural anesthesia include the use of anticoagulant or antiplatelet medications in the case of bleeding tendency, lack of patient cooperation, skin infection at the puncture site, and intracranial hypertension. In children, epidural anesthesia may be performed after induction of general anesthesia but should be performed by a skilled anesthesiologist.

Catheter malposition in the subarachnoid space or a vein has been reported during epidural anesthesia, not only at the time of puncture but also at any point in the postoperative period [13], and while confirmation with a test dose at the time of puncture is performed as a matter of course, continuous observation of the general condition is also necessary in the postoperative ward.

During surgery, a high concentration of local anesthetic may be used intentionally to relieve tension in the abdominal wall and to provide some muscle relaxant effect. Residual muscle weakness in the lower extremities may remain even after the end of the surgery, and the patient should be made aware of this when being transferred from the operating room. This is because it is necessary to distinguish this from the above-mentioned catheter malposition in the subarachnoid space. One should also suspect local anesthetic toxicity if dysgeusia or polyphrasia appears. Epidural hematoma and abscess are also complications that require attention, and if back pain or muscle weakness in the lower extremities lead to a suspicion of such complications, MRI imaging should be performed promptly.

If anesthetic effect is inadequate, a cold test should be performed, the number of times the PCA button is pressed should be checked, and the catheter position should be confirmed. Based on this information, the bolus dose amount and continuous dose amount may be increased, and the catheter position may be adjusted to obtain adequate anesthetic effect and extent. Currently, postoperative pain management teams consisting of anesthesiologists, scrub nurses, and pharmacists are evaluating and improving postoperative pain management, but there are large differences among facilities in how effectively this is being implemented.

8. Advantages of analgesic administration by intravenous (IV) PCA

The analgesia by intravenous administration of opioids is superior in that the route of administration is easy to establish, and the onset of effect is rapid. When used for postoperative analgesia, IV-PCA should be connected after maintaining a certain concentration in the blood by the time the patient awakens from anesthesia. Fentanyl is often used, but morphine is more common worldwide. Because of the short duration of effect of fentanyl, IV-PCA with continuous administration of fentanyl is often used, and one should watch for sedation and respiratory depression. Considering that postoperative pain decreases over time, continuously administered fentanyl should be tapered off over time. Patients should be advised that a single bolus dose of PCA is unlikely to relieve severe pain and that they should not tolerate pain but should press the PCA button "at the point of onset of pain" or "at the point one feels uncomfortable." As has been mentioned earlier, it is important to note that acetaminophen and nonsteroidal anti-inflammatory drugs (NSAIDs) are available as basal analgesics.

Administration of narcotics also increases postoperative nausea and vomiting (PONV). PONV on the day following surgery is as high as 6.9% in the epidural anesthesia group versus 21.6% in the IV-PCA group [14], suggesting the active use of antiemetics so that PONV does not hinder early mobilization.

Drug addiction has become a problem in the United States. In the United States, in patients who become chronic drug users after surgery, an association was found between the patient behavior and pain disorder [15]. It is now clear that patients with a predisposition become chronic users of easily prescribed opioids following surgery, regardless of whether the surgery is major or minor, and that careless prescribing of opioids should be discouraged. In particular, respiratory depression can be fatal in obese patients and patients with chronic obstructive pulmonary disease and sleep apnea. Opioid-free anesthesia [16, 17] has proven effective for such patients.

9. Advantages of peripheral nerve block

In recent years, the launch of a series of echo machines that allow for more detailed checks has made it possible to administer local anesthesia or place a catheter after confirming the nerve during peripheral nerve blocks. In the past, local anesthesia was often administered blindly using a blood vessel or bone as a landmark or by attaching a nerve stimulator to the needle tip and administering local anesthesia where the needle tip felt a muscle contraction, which could lead to inadequate effect or complications from blood vessel or direct nerve puncture. Now that the nerves can be seen directly, nerve blocks can be performed more peripherally and only where necessary. Since nerve blocks can be performed at any site where blood flow can be stopped from the surface of the body, even while the patient is on anticoagulants, there are fewer restrictions based on the patient's condition.

10. Program for enhanced recovery after surgery

To help patients undergoing surgery to recover fast and be discharged from the hospital, perioperative management through a program for enhanced recovery after surgery, known as ERAS (Enhanced Recovery After Surgery), has been implemented in Europe [18–24]. This is a multidisciplinary program that includes postoperative pain management, early mobilization, and early oral intake. The program started in 1999 with a report that postoperative hospital stay for sigmoid colon resection was reduced from the previous 5–10 days to a median of 2 days [25]. Since then, the European Society for Clinical Nutrition and Metabolism has taken the lead in promoting the use of this program, and many studies were conducted to review the timing of preoperative oral intake, bowel preparation, and the start of postoperative oral intake. The program places importance on the team approach to healthcare, in which preoperative, intraoperative, and postoperative management is seamlessly carried out through multidisciplinary collaboration. Furthermore, being up-to-date is what makes this program appealing; for example, epidural anesthesia for laparotomy, which was strongly promoted at the beginning, is no longer strongly recommended for routine surgeries [21, 24], and multimodal analgesia is now being considered, which combines the use of wound infusion catheter and subarachnoid opioids and so on.

11. Delirium

Generally, muscle weakness occurs at a rate of about 1–3% per day or 10–15% per week while the patient remains at bed rest and is said to deteriorate to 50% in 3–5 weeks. Muscle weakness can easily lead to frailty and sarcopenia in the elderly. Development of postoperative delirium is a major obstacle in the implementation of the ERAS program and early discharge from the hospital. Postoperative delirium is a serious postoperative complication that prolongs hospital stay and worsens prognosis [26, 27]. Postoperative delirium can also cause postoperative cognitive decline [28] and threatens subsequent social life. It has been reported that 80% of elderly patients develop postoperative delirium while in the intensive care unit (ICU) [29]. Postoperative delirium occurs in the elderly and is also associated with brain vulnerability. Factors contributing to delirium can be divided into (1) predisposing factors, (2) triggering factors, and (3) direct factors. Predisposing factors include advanced age, dementia, alcoholism or polydipsia, and history of psychiatric illness. Triggering factors include psychological stress, ICU stay, sleep deprivation, and postoperative pain. Direct factors include dehydration, infection, and electrolyte imbalance. Despite screening based on risk factors at the time of admission, focused care of patients prone to delirium, environmental modification, and elimination of causes, delirium still develops at a high rate in the elderly. Pharmacotherapy using psychoactive drugs is given for symptomatic treatment. Haloperidol, quetiapine, and risperidone are used [30]. However, there is no evidence of efficacy of these psychoactive drugs with respect to duration and severity of delirium, length of hospitalization, and mortality [31].

There are numerous reports on the efficacy of dexmedetomidine in the prevention and treatment of delirium [32–34]. New sleep medications, ramelteon and suvorexant, have also been reported to have preventive and therapeutic effects [35–37] and are increasingly prescribed on regular basis rather than as-needed. At our institution, we hypothesized that heart-rate variability could be used to predict delirium, and we have found that changes in autonomic nerves on the day before surgery can help predict delirium [38].

12. Conclusion

As surgeries with small incision are becoming mainstream, early discharge following the ERAS protocol is beneficial for the medical economics as well as for the patient's life. Methods of anesthesia that use anesthetics with minimal side effects and no postoperative residual effect, that provide sufficient postoperative analgesia, and that do not interfere with early mobilization are desirable. Elderly patients are also proactively undergoing surgery, and we hope that they get through the perioperative period smoothly and fully enjoy a 100-year-lifespan.

Acknowledgements

This work was supported by Grants-in-Aid for Scientific Research (KAKENHI) Grants No. 19 K18308 and No. 22 K09081.

Conflict of interest

The authors declare no conflict of interest.

Author details

Maiko Satomoto
Department of Anesthesiology, Toho University Omori Medical Center, Tokyo, Japan

*Address all correspondence to: maiko.satomoto@med.toho-u.ac.jp

References

[1] Ready LB, Oden R, Chadwick HS, Benedetti C, Rooke GA, Caplan R, et al. Development of an anesthesiology-based postoperative pain management service. Anesthesiology. 1988;**68**:100-106. DOI: 10.1097/00000542-198801000-00016

[2] Werner MU, Søholm L, Rotbøll-Nielsen P, Kehlet H. Does an acute pain service improve postoperative outcome? Anesthesia and Analgesia. 2002;**95**:1361-1372. DOI: 10.1097/00000539-200211000-00049

[3] Kehlet H, Jensen TS, Woolf CJ. Persistent postsurgical pain: Risk factors and prevention. Lancet. 2006;**367**:1618-1625. DOI: 10.1016/S0140-6736(06)68700-X

[4] Nikolajsen L, Ilkjaer S, Krøner K, Christensen JH, Jensen TS. The influence of preamputation pain on postamputation stump and phantom pain. Pain. 1997;**72**:393-405. DOI: 10.1016/s0304-3959(97)00061-4

[5] Tasmuth T, Estlanderb AM, Kalso E. Effect of present pain and mood on the memory of past postoperative pain in women treated surgically for breast cancer. Pain. 1996;**68**:343-347. DOI: 10.1016/s0304-3959(96)03219-8

[6] Katz J, Jackson M, Kavanagh BP, Sandler AN. Acute pain after thoracic surgery predicts long-term post-thoracotomy pain. The Clinical Journal of Pain. 1996;**12**(1):50-55. DOI: 10.1097/00002508-199603000-00009

[7] Chou R, Gordon DB, de Leon-Casasola OA, Rosenberg JM, Bickler S, Brennan T, et al. Management of Postoperative Pain: A Clinical Practice Guideline from the American Pain Society, the American Society of Regional Anesthesia and Pain Medicine, and the American Society of Anesthesiologists' Committee on Regional Anesthesia, Executive Committee, and Administrative Council. The Journal of Pain. 2016;**17**:131-157. DOI: 10.1016/j.jpain.2015.12.008

[8] Roofthooft E, Joshi GP, Rawal N, Van de Velde M, PROSPECT Working Group* of the European Society of Regional Anaesthesia and Pain Therapy and supported by the Obstetric Anaesthetists' Association. PROSPECT guideline for elective caesarean section: Updated systematic review and procedure-specific postoperative pain management recommendations. Anaesthesia. 2021;**76**:665-680. DOI: 10.1111/anae.15339

[9] Anger M, Valovska T, Beloeil H, Lirk P, Joshi GP, Van de Velde M, et al. PROSPECT guideline for total hip arthroplasty: A systematic review and procedure-specific postoperative pain management recommendations. Anaesthesia. 2021;**76**:1082-1097. DOI: 10.1111/anae.15498

[10] Barazanchi AWH, MacFater WS, Rahiri JL, Tutone S, Hill AG, Joshi GP. PROSPECT collaboration. Evidence-based management of pain after laparoscopic cholecystectomy: A PROSPECT review update. British Journal of Anaesthesia. 2018;**121**:787-803. DOI: 10.1016/j.bja.2018.06.023

[11] Lemoine A, Witdouck A, Beloeil H, Bonnet F, PROSPECT Working Group of the European Society of Regional Anaesthesia and Pain Therapy (ESRA). PROSPECT guidelines update for evidence-based pain management after prostatectomy for cancer.

Anaesthia Critical Care Pain Medicine. 2021;**40**:100922. DOI: 10.1016/j.accpm.2021.100922

[12] Lirk P, Thiry J, Bonnet MP, Joshi GP, Bonnet F, PROSPECT Working Group. Pain management after laparoscopic hysterectomy: Systematic review of literature and PROSPECT recommendations. Regional Anesthesia and Pain Medicine. 2019;**44**:425-436. DOI: 10.1136/rapm-2018-100024

[13] Matunaga M, Tsuchimochi H, Ikeda S, Hara H, Shono S, Higa K. Profound sedation and subarachnoid migration of an epidural catheter : A report of two cases. Journal of Japan Society of Pain Clinicians (JJSPC). 2005;**12**:29-32. DOI: 10.11321/jjspc 1994.12.29

[14] Hamada H. Safe and efficient postoperative pain management. The Journal of Japan Society for Clinical Anesthesia. 2017;**37**:49-57. DOI: 10.2199/jjsca.37.49

[15] Brummett CM, Waljee JF, Goesling J, Moser S, Lin P, Englesbe MJ, et al. New persistent opioid use after minor and major surgical procedures in US adults. JAMA Surgery. 2017;**152**:e170504. DOI: 10.1001/jamasurg.2017.0504

[16] Boysen PG, Pappas MM, Evans B. An evidence-based opioid-free Anesthetic technique to manage perioperative and periprocedural pain. The Ochsner Journal. 2018;**18**:121-125. DOI: 10.31486/toj.17.0072

[17] Sultana A, Torres D, Schumann R. Special indications for opioid free anaesthesia and analgesia, patient and procedure related: Including obesity, sleep apnoea, chronic obstructive pulmonary disease, complex regional pain syndromes, opioid addiction and cancer surgery. Best Practise Research Clinical Anaesthesiology. 2017;**31**:547-560. DOI: 10.1016/j.bpa.2017.11.002

[18] Lassen K, Soop M, Nygren J, Cox PB, Hendry PO, Spies C, et al. Consensus review of optimal perioperative care in colorectal surgery: Enhanced Recovery After Surgery (ERAS) Group recommendations. Achieves in Surgery. 2009;**144**:961-969. DOI: 10.1001/archsurg.2009.170

[19] Wainwright TW, Gill M, McDonald DA, Middleton RG, Reed M, Sahota O, et al. Consensus statement for perioperative care in total hip replacement and total knee replacement surgery: Enhanced Recovery After Surgery (ERAS®) Society recommendations. Acta Orthopaedica. 2020;**91**:3-19. DOI: 10.1080/17453674.2019.1683790

[20] Debono B, Wainwright TW, Wang MY, Sigmundsson FG, Yang MMH, Smid-Nanninga H, et al. Consensus statement for perioperative care in lumbar spinal fusion: Enhanced Recovery After Surgery (ERAS®) society recommendations. The Spine Journal. 2021;**21**:729-752. DOI: 10.1016/j.spinee.2021.01.001

[21] Gustafsson UO, Scott MJ, Hubner M, Nygren J, Demartines N, Francis N, et al. Guidelines for perioperative Care in Elective Colorectal Surgery: Enhanced Recovery After Surgery (ERAS®) society recommendations: 2018. World Journal of Surgery. 2019;**43**:659-695. DOI: 10.1007/s00268-018-4844-y

[22] Temple-Oberle C, Shea-Budgell MA, Tan M, Semple JL, Schrag C, Barreto M, et al. Consensus review of optimal perioperative Care in Breast Reconstruction: Enhanced Recovery after Surgery (ERAS) society recommendations. Plastic and Reconstructive Surgery.

2017;**139**:1056e-1071e. DOI: 10.1097/PRS.0000000000003242

[23] Batchelor TJP, Rasburn NJ, Abdelnour-Berchtold E, Brunelli A, Cerfolio RJ, Gonzalez M, et al. Guidelines for enhanced recovery after lung surgery: Recommendations of the Enhanced Recovery After Surgery (ERAS®) society and the European Society of Thoracic Surgeons (ESTS). European Journal of Cardio-Thoracic Surgery. 2019;**55**:91-115. DOI: 10.1093/ejcts/ezy301

[24] Melloul E, Hübner M, Scott M, Snowden C, Prentis J, Dejong CH, et al. Guidelines for perioperative care for liver surgery: Enhanced Recovery After Surgery (ERAS) Society Recommendations. World Journal of Surgery. 2016;**40**:2425-2440. DOI: 10.1007/s00268-016-3700-1

[25] Kehlet H, Mogensen T. Hospital stay of 2 days after open sigmoidectomy with a multimodal rehabilitation programme. The British Journal of Surgery. 1999;**86**:227-230. DOI: 10.1046/j.1365-2168.1999.01023.x

[26] Leslie DL, Zhang Y, Holford TR, Bogardus ST, Leo-Summers LS, Inouye SK. Premature death associated with delirium at 1-year follow-up. Archives of Internal Medicine. 2005;**165**:1657-1662. DOI: 10.1001/archinte.165.14.1657

[27] National Clinical Guideline Centre (UK). Delirium: Diagnosis, Prevention and Management. London: Royal College of Physicians (UK); 2010

[28] Huang H, Li H, Zhang X, Shi G, Xu M, Ru X, et al. Association of postoperative delirium with cognitive outcomes: A meta-analysis. Journal of Clinical Anesthesiology. 2021;**75**:110496. DOI: 10.1016/j.jclinane.2021.110496

[29] Girard TD, Ware LB, Bernard GR, et al. Associations of markers of inflammation and coagulation with delirium during critical illness. Intensive Care Medicine. 2012;**38**:1965-1973. DOI: 10.1007/s00134-012-2678-x

[30] Okumura Y, Hatta K, Wada K, Takeuchi T, Kishi Y, DELIRIA-J Group. Expert opinions on the first-line pharmacological treatment for delirium in Japan: A conjoint analysis. International Psychogeriatrics. 2016;**28**:1041-1050. DOI: 10.1017/S1041610215002446

[31] Siddiqi N, Harrison JK, Clegg A, Teale EA, Young J, Taylor J, et al. Interventions for preventing delirium in hospitalised non-ICU patients. Cochrane Database of Systematic Reviews. 2016;**3**:CD005563. DOI: 10.1002/14651858.CD005563.pub3

[32] Mo Y, Zimmermann AE. Role of dexmedetomidine for the prevention and treatment of delirium in intensive care unit patients. The Annals of Pharmacotherapy. 2013;**47**:869-876. DOI: 10.1345/aph.1AR708

[33] Xia ZQ, Chen SQ, Yao X, Xie CB, Wen SH, Liu KX. Clinical benefits of dexmedetomidine versus propofol in adult intensive care unit patients: A meta-analysis of randomized clinical trials. The Journal of Surgical Research. 2013;**185**:833-843. DOI: 10.1016/j.jss.2013.06.062

[34] Deiner S, Luo X, Lin HM, Sessler DI, Saager L, Sieber FE, et al. Intraoperative infusion of Dexmedetomidine for prevention of postoperative delirium and cognitive dysfunction in elderly patients undergoing major elective noncardiac surgery: A randomized clinical trial. JAMA Surgery. 2017;**152**:e171505. DOI: 10.1001/jamasurg.2017.1505

[35] Hatta K, Kishi Y, Wada K, Takeuchi T, Ito S, Kurata A, et al. Preventive effects of Suvorexant on delirium: A randomized placebo-controlled trial. The Journal of Clinical Psychiatry. 2017;**78**:e970-e979. DOI: 10.4088/JCP.16m11194

[36] Hatta K, Kishi Y, Wada K, Takeuchi T, Odawara T, Usui C, et al. Preventive effects of ramelteon on delirium: A randomized placebo-controlled trial. JAMA Psychiatry. 2014;**71**:397-403. DOI: 10.1001/jamapsychiatry.2013.3320

[37] Hatta K, Kishi Y, Wada K, Takeuchi T, Hashimoto N, Suda K, et al. Real-world effectiveness of Ramelteon and Suvorexant for delirium prevention in 948 patients with delirium risk factors. The Journal of Clinical Psychiatry. 2019;**81**:19m12865. DOI: 10.4088/JCP.19m12865

[38] Echizen M, Satomoto M, Miyajima M, Adachi Y, Matsushima E. Preoperative heart rate variability analysis is as a potential simple and easy measure for predicting perioperative delirium in esophageal surgery. Annals of Meical Surgery (Lond). 2021;**70**:102856. DOI: 10.1016/j.amsu.2021.102856

Chapter 3

Enhanced Recovery after Surgery

Navin Kumar, Rohik Anjum, Dhiraj Mallik, Farhanul Huda, Bibek Karki and Somprakas Basu

Abstract

Enhanced recovery after surgery (ERAS) protocols are specialized perioperative care guidelines. The protocol was first published in 2005. Since then, it has been associated with improved perioperative outcomes. This multimodal peri-operative protocols standardize the perioperative care to minimize the surgical stress response and post-operative pain, reduce complications, improve post-operative outcomes, expedite recovery and decrease the length of hospital stay. It initially started with colorectal surgery, but now it is used in hepatobiliary, upper gastrointestinal system, urology, gynecology, vascular surgery, bariatric, and non-gastro intestinal specialties. Its role is well established in elective surgery. Now there are enough evidence suggesting its role in emergency surgeries as well. There are 24 elements of the ERAS bundle. However, only some critical elements of the ERAS bundle are feasible to be used in emergency surgery. Postoperative pain management is one of the significant elements in the ERAS bundle. Multimodal analgesia is the optimal modality for pain control. It facilitates early ambulation and rehabilitation. Current evidence recommends the ERAS protocol. However, each item within the protocol constantly changes over time, depending upon the evidence.

Keywords: ERAS, length of hospital stay, postoperative pain, perioperative care, protocol, multimodal analgesia

1. Introduction

There are various challenges in the care of a patient in his surgical journey, which starts from preadmission, preoperative, and intraoperative care till postoperative recovery. Each unit has its focus, affecting the one to follow. The same surgery may have different outcomes because the surgical outcome depends on the perioperative management rather than the actual operation. Patients require hospital care after major abdominal surgery because of the need for parenteral analgesia for persistent pain and intravenous fluid because of bowel dysfunction and postoperative complications. The length of hospital stay may vary in different parts of the world because of the variation in perioperative care. Henrik Kehlet showed that a patient could be discharged in 2 days after the open sigmoid resections [1]. The length of stay after these operations was ten days in most countries; thus, he pioneered fast-track surgery [2].

In earlier days, postoperative care was different among different centers because of the lack of specific protocols for specific organ-based surgeries. It was decided to promote the change in practice in the care of surgical patients. The Enhanced

Recovery After Surgery (ERAS) study group was formed in 2001 in Europe to combat this problem. Professor Ken Fearon, University of Edinburgh, UK, and Professor Olle Ljungqvist, Karolinska Institute, Sweden, assembled in 2001 to develop ideas about ERAS with the surgical department or Universities of three other northern European Countries (Denmark, Norway, and The Netherlands) [3]. They found a discrepancy between the actual practices and evidence-based best practices. Much published evidence suggests that perioperative care differs in different parts of the world, and there is a minimum adherence to evidence-based practice [4].

The aim of the ERAS study group (http://www.erassociety.org) was to find out the ways for quality surgical recovery rather than speed. The study group met several times to reach a consensus on a protocol to improve the quality of surgical recovery. These were called ERAS protocols. These are procedure-specific guidelines. The group focused on enhancing recovery and reducing complications by modifying the metabolic response to surgical insult rather than limiting the length of stay. They found that early mobilization and enteral nutrition are beneficial in the postoperative period, leading to rapid hospital discharge [5]. The first guideline was published in 2005 for colorectal surgery [3]. In 2012 the guidelines were divided into colonic and rectal surgery, but in 2018 these two surgical specialties guidelines were combined [6–8]. The Dutch group led the implementation of the first guidelines and showed improvements in recovery time [9]. They showed that the guidelines could be implemented in a structured way. ERAS protocol, when implemented in a structured way, showed a significant reduction in postoperative morbidity (48%) and length of hospital stay (2.5 days) in colorectal surgery when compared with traditional perioperative care [10, 11]. The ERAS society was registered in Sweden in 2010 (www.erassociety.org). This is an international non-profit medical academic society whose members are from different professions involved in surgical care [5].

Current evidence recommends the ERAS protocol as a whole (all elements) and not as a single element. However, each element within the protocol constantly changes over time, depending upon the evidence. Now, these protocols have been adapted for the upper gastrointestinal system, urology, gynecology, vascular surgery, hepato-pancreatico-biliary, esophageal, bariatric, and non-gastrointestinal specialties [12, 13]. The ERAS guideline has changed over the years since its inception. The first ERAS guideline was based on expert opinion and literature review, but the recent guideline is based on evidence-based grading.

2. Components of ERAS

There are 24 components of ERAS that are used by different surgical specialties of the hospital for different patients (**Table 1**) [8].

2.1 Preadmission

2.1.1 Preadmission information, education, and counseling

It is recommended that proper preoperative counseling should be done as it not only takes out the fear of surgery but also helps in pain control to a reasonable amount which ultimately will lead to an early discharge for the patient [14–18]. Patient education via leaflets, drawings, and multimedia (like various videos) of the surgical

ERAS item	
1	Preadmission information, education, and counseling
2	Preoperative optimization
3	Prehabilitation
4	Preoperative nutritional care
5	Management of anemia
6	Prevention of nausea and vomiting
7	Pre-anesthetic medication
8	Antimicrobial prophylaxis and skin preparation
9	Bowel preparation
10	Preoperative fluid and electrolyte therapy
11	Preoperative fasting and carbohydrate loading
12	Standard anesthetic protocol
13	Intraoperative fluid and electrolyte therapy
14	Preventing intraoperative hypothermia
15	Surgical access (open and minimally invasive surgery including laparoscopic, robotic, and trans-anal approaches)
16	Drainage of peritoneal cavity and pelvis
17	Nasogastric intubation
18	Postoperative analgesia
19	thromboprophylaxis
20	Postoperative fluid and electrolyte therapy
21	Urinary drainage
22	Prevention of postoperative ileus
23	Postoperative glycaemic control
24	Postoperative nutritional care

Table 1.
ERAS guidelines 2018 for colorectal surgery (http://www.erassociety.org) [8].

procedures also improves pain and anxiety after surgery. Patients should always be designated a particular role post-surgery, including proper nutrition and mobilization [14, 19, 20]. The grade of recommendation is strong.

2.1.2 Preoperative optimization: (risk assessment, abstinence of smoking and alcohol)

Preoperative risk assessment of the patient should be done along with optimization of heart, lung, and kidney diseases, diabetes, hypertension, anemia, malnutrition, and cessation of excessive alcohol and smoking. Smokers have an increased risk of intraoperative and postoperative complications [21]. Counseling and nicotine replacement are very effective methods in preoperative smoking cessation [22]. At least 4–8 weeks of abstinence is required to reduce respiratory and wound healing complications [23, 24]. Alcohol abuse increases postoperative morbidity but not mortality. At least four weeks of abstinence is required [25]. The grade of recommendation for preoperative optimization is strong.

2.1.3 Prehabilitation

Prehabilitation is the period between diagnosis and the beginning of acute treatment. It is done to improve the physical and psychological health of the patient. Poor preoperative physical health is a risk factor for postoperative complications. Its grade of recommendation is weak.

2.1.4 Preoperative nutritional care

A preoperative nutritional assessment should be done to detect malnutrition. In malnourished patients, enteral or additional parenteral nutrition should be added 7–10 days preoperatively. It reduces infectious complications and anastomotic leaks [26]. Its grade of recommendation is strong.

2.1.5 Management of anemia

Anemia is the risk factor for morbidity and mortality, and blood transfusion also increases complications. A 60-100 g/L of Hb should be maintained before surgery [27]. Its grade of recommendation is strong.

2.2 Preoperative items

2.2.1 Postoperative nausea and vomiting

Postoperative nausea and vomiting (PONV) are important causes of patient dissatisfaction. PONV affects 30–50% of patients [28]. The etiology of PONV is multifactorial. Prophylactic treatment should be given to prevent postoperative nausea and vomiting. There are several scoring systems for predicting a risk factor for PONV. Koivuranta and Apfel's scoring system is most commonly used [29–31]. A multimodal approach should be considered to prevent PONV. Patients with 1–2 risk factors should be given a two-drug combination as prophylactic antiemetics, whereas 2–3 antiemetics should be given in patients with >2 risk factors. Its grade of recommendation is strong.

2.2.2 Pre-anesthetic medication

A high level of anxiety occurs in the perioperative period, which increases the analgesic requirements and postoperative complications. Anxiolytic should be given to decrease the psychological stress, which subsequently decreases the perioperative analgesic requirement [32]. Its grade of recommendation is strong.

2.2.3 Antimicrobial and skin preparation

Intravenous antibiotic prophylaxis should be given 60 minutes prior to the incision. There is a reduction in surgical site infection (SSI) after oral and systemic antibiotics, along with mechanical bowel preparation in colorectal surgery. The SSI rate further decreases after skin decontamination with chlorhexidine. Although preoperative hair removal does not decrease SSI incidence, it should preferably be performed using clippers [33]. The grade of recommendation is strong for intravenous antibiotic prophylaxis and skin decontamination by chlorhexidine.

2.2.4 Preoperative fluid and electrolyte therapy

Preoperative fluid and electrolyte deficits should be corrected before the patient reaches the operating room. Its grade of recommendation is strong.

2.2.5 Preoperative fasting and carbohydrate loading

Old school thought of prolonged fasting before major surgeries are being taken out of recommendations. Nowadays, light meals can be taken 6 hours prior to induction while clear liquids, specifically carbohydrate drinks (a 12-ounce clear beverage or a 24-g complex carbohydrate beverage), 2 hours prior to induction [34]. Evidence shows that it decreases dehydration and hypotension intraoperatively and also decreases insulin resistance, thus enhancing postoperative metabolism [35]. The grade of recommendation is strong.

2.3 Intraoperative components

2.3.1 Standard anesthetic protocol

Benzodiazepines should be avoided, and short-acting anesthetic agents should be used. Propofol should be used for induction of anesthesia. It can be combined with short-acting opioids such as fentanyl, alfentanil, sufentanil or remifentanil infusions. This minimizes residual effects at the end of anesthesia. This will allow rapid reversal [8]. Cerebral monitoring should be done to reduce the risk of delirium.

2.3.2 Intraoperative fluid and electrolyte therapy

Fluid management is crucial to maintaining intravascular volume, cardiac output, and tissue perfusion. The main aim is to reduce the hydrostatic pressure in pulmonary capillaries. Before ERAS, there was a restriction in fluid management where the rate for maintenance fluid was 1-2 ml/kg/hr., with perioperative fluid being <1500 ml or 20 ml/kg/24 hrs. In ERAS protocol, it is always a goal-directed therapy (GTD) for fluids, which reduces postoperative morbidity and decreases the length of stay in the hospital. Now balanced crystalloids at a rate of 1-4 ml/kg/hour are the fluid of choice over 0.9% normal saline (NS) but should be discontinued postoperatively. Again, liberal fluid management can also harm the patient postoperatively by intestinal edema and delayed return of bowel movements [36].

2.3.3 Preventing intraoperative hypothermia

Normothermia should be maintained throughout the surgery. This can be done by warming and humidifying anesthetic gases and warming intravenous and irrigation fluids.

2.3.4 Drainage of the peritoneal cavity and pelvis

Many published studies do not support the use of the intraperitoneal drain. It has no effect on clinical outcomes and should not be used routinely. The grade of recommendation is strong.

2.4 Postoperative items

2.4.1 Nasogastric intubation

Its aim was to reduce postoperative gastric distension and vomiting. A Cochrane meta-analysis does not support it. It should be used sparingly. If inserted intraoperatively, it should be removed before anesthesia reversal [37, 38].

2.4.2 Anesthesia and pain relief

In line with ERAS protocol, pain relief is a multimodal approach that uses regional anesthesia. It avoids the use of opioids. Relief from postoperative pain decreases immediate risks of hypoxemia, hypercarbia, increased myocardial work, arrhythmias, and ischemia. Therefore, enhanced recovery pathways must combine multimodal enteral and parenteral analgesia with regional analgesia or local anesthetic techniques. It should also be kept in mind that the impact of an anesthetic agent on organ function should be minimum. Depth of anesthesia should be appropriate to avoid an overdose. It is better to use short-acting agents than total intravenous anesthesia.

Postoperative pain is one of the most important reasons for immobilization, delayed oral intake, and prolonged hospital stay. Therefore, to avoid these, the protective role of epidural analgesia has become an essential element in ERAS protocol. It mainly reduces stress hormones secretion and insulin resistance. Usually, an epidural catheter is inserted just before the induction or during surgery; either a continuous infusion (4–10 ml/hr) or intermittent top-up of a local anesthetic agent (bupivacaine 0.1%) can be given along with a low dose of opioid (to avoid opioid related systemic side effects) via the epidural catheter. Usually, the catheter is kept for two days. No other mode of analgesia is required during this duration, and using another analgesic during those two days is not recommended.

Apart from this, there are other modalities for pain relief, such as paravertebral block, serratus anterior plane block, rectus abdominis block, and transversus abdominis block. However, all these are less proven for pain relief than epidural analgesia [39].

The surgical aspect of ERAS in pain relief is equally important for a better postoperative recovery. Prolonged and open surgeries hamper postoperative mobilization, pain control, and oral intake and even increase the length of hospital stay. Thus, minimally invasive approaches are recommended for their effectiveness in reducing postoperative complications, including hospital stays. It is seen that less tissue handling during surgery improves postoperative recovery [40].

Apart from epidural analgesia, enteral analgesics are also recommended to reduce pain, postoperative nausea, vomiting, and the start of oral feeds. Enteral analgesics that can be used are acetaminophen (most commonly) and NSAIDs (avoided in renal failure, Diabetic patients, and old age patients) [35]. For the facilitation of pain management protocol in ERAS, a PROSPECT (PROcedure-SPEcific Postoperative Pain Management) working group was constituted. This collaboration provides evidence-based, procedure-specific pain management recommendations (www.postoppain.org) [41, 42]. This approach improved compliance with pain management recommendations in an ERAS bundle.

2.4.3 Thromboprophylaxis

Mechanical thromboprophylaxis and compression stockings or intermittent pneumatic compression should be advised to all high-risk surgical patients undergoing major surgery (malignancy, hypercoagulable state, steroid use, advanced age, and obesity) [43–45]. Mechanical thromboprophylaxis should be continued until discharge.

2.4.4 Postoperative fluid and electrolyte therapy

ERAS states that it should be neither restrictive nor liberal in giving fluid therapy both intraoperatively and postoperatively. Maintenance fluid should always be given according to the body weight, with supplementing electrolytes over 24 hrs. Too much fluid might lead to intestinal edema, resulting in decreased bowel movement and delayed oral intake. Thus increasing postoperative complications and increased length of hospital stay [46]. The patient should be encouraged to oral liquids when they are awake.

2.4.5 Urinary drainage

Urinary catheterization can cause urinary tract infection (UTI), which is directly related to the duration of catheterization. So, the duration of catheterization should be individualized based on the risk factor of urinary retention (male gender, epidural anesthesia, pelvic surgery). In low-risk cases catheter should be removed on the first day of surgery, whereas in high risk, it should be kept for up to 3 days.

2.4.6 Prevention of postoperative ileus

It is a significant cause of postoperative discomfort and length of hospital stay. The ERAS items, like limiting the use of opioids and encouraging the use of multimodal analgesia, minimally invasive surgery, avoiding routine nasogastric tube insertion, and maintaining goal-directed fluid therapy, can limit the postoperative ileus [6].

2.4.7 Postoperative glycaemic control

The physiological response to surgical injury is insulin resistance which can persist for several weeks after elective surgery [47]. Hyperglycaemia is a risk factor for surgery. This can be prevented in the ERAS pathway by giving preoperative oral carbohydrate loading, laparoscopic surgery, and epidural analgesia.

2.4.8 Postoperative nutritional care

Early oral feeds are another essential element in ERAS protocol that reduces postoperative complications (postoperative ileus) and length of hospital stay. It also helps reduce any in-hospital infection. Studies have shown that there is no advantage in keeping nil by mouth for patients undergoing major surgeries, which instead hampers fast recovery. However, patients with early oral feeds are also at risk of nausea and vomiting. To prevent this, a targeted strategy should be planned. Use of anti-emetic drugs to be adopted and emetogenic drugs (opioids) should be avoided [48].

2.4.9 Early mobilization

Postoperatively patient has to mobilize as early as possible to avoid pulmonary complications, reduced muscle strength, risk of thromboembolism, insulin resistance, delayed bowel movements, and prolonged hospital stay [19].

3. ERAS in emergency surgery

This has been proven that ERAS has a defined role in elective surgery [49]. However, the effectiveness of these protocols in emergency abdominal surgeries has been nominally studied. The protocols that have been clearly defined for elective surgeries were not fully applicable in emergency surgeries, and there would be difficulty in compliance with the set protocols. However, some elements of the ERAS bundle can be included in emergency surgeries. The recent evidence showed a reduced length of stay and postoperative complications on implementing even tailored ERAS protocols in emergency abdominal surgeries [50]. Tailoring of the ERAS protocol can be done to include only critical items which can facilitate program implementation in emergency surgery. This has shown better outcomes and a reduction in the cost of care in emergency surgery. Recent studies have shown that 70% of the ERAS bundle is required to get the beneficial effects [51–53].

4. Impact of ERAS

ERAS is described as an intention to treat analysis. The compliance rate of ERAS may vary which depends on different surgical approaches and diseases. Minimally invasive surgery with minimal tubes and drains is considered a standard of care.

Postoperative pain management is one of the major elements in the ERAS bundle. It facilitates early ambulation and rehabilitation, ultimately reducing length of hospital stay [41, 54]. Inadequate postoperative pain relief may lead to chronic pain development and ultimately increase the readmission rate [54, 55]. The ERAS protocols reduce the length of hospital stay (3–5 days) as well as a significant reduction in overall morbidity (Relative Risk of 0.6,95% CI 0.46–0.76), without any higher readmission rate [56]. In addition to reduced length of hospital stay and morbidity, there is enhanced recovery, including reduced duration of ileus, preservation of lean body mass, and a more active lifestyle [57].

5. Conclusion

Enhanced recovery after surgery (ERAS) are specially designed multimodal perioperative care pathways for a speedy recovery. ERAS pathways are the standard of care, but their widespread dissemination is still challenging. Some elements of the ERAS bundle, like minimally invasive surgery and limiting tubes and drains, are standard of care and are being followed in most of the centers. However, the other elements of the ERAS bundle, like preoperative carbohydrate loading and postoperative early ambulation, still need to be implemented in routine clinical practice. There is considerable difficulty in adherence to the complete ERAS bundle. Postoperative pain management is one of the major elements in the ERAS bundle. Multimodal analgesia is the optimal modality for pain control. It facilitates early ambulation and rehabilitation. It also decreases the duration of ileus and morbidity, ultimately reducing the hospital stay and readmission rate. Current evidence recommends ERAS protocol as a whole and not as a few elements within it. However, each item within the protocol constantly changes over time, depending upon the evidence.

Conflict of interest

The authors declare no conflict of interest.

Author details

Navin Kumar*, Rohik Anjum, Dhiraj Mallik, Farhanul Huda, Bibek Karki and Somprakas Basu
Department of Surgery, All India Institute of Medical Sciences, Rishikesh, India

*Address all correspondence to: navin.surg@aiimsrishikesh.edu.in

References

[1] Kehlet H. Multimodal approach to control postoperative pathophysiology and rehabilitation. British Journal of Anaesthesia. 1997;**78**:606-617

[2] Kehlet H, Mogensen T. Hospital stay of 2 days after open sigmoidectomy with a multimodal rehabilitation programme. The British Journal of Surgery. 1999;**86**:227-230

[3] Fearon KC, Ljungqvist O, Von Meyenfeldt M, et al. Enhanced recovery after surgery: A consensus review of clinical care for patients undergoing colonic resection. Clinical Nutrition. 2005;**24**(3):466-477

[4] Lassen K, Hannemann P, Ljungqvist O, et al. Enhanced recovery after surgery group. Patterns in current perioperative practice: Survey of colorectal surgeons in five northern European countries. BMJ. 2005;**330**(7505):1420-1421

[5] Ljungqvist O, Young-Fadok T, Demartines N. The history of enhanced recovery after surgery and the ERAS society. Journal of Laparoendoscopic & Advanced Surgical Techniques. Part A. 2017;**27**:860-862

[6] Gustafsson UO, Scott MJ, Schwenk W, et al. Guidelines for perioperative care in elective colonic surgery: Enhanced recovery after surgery (ERAS(®)) society recommendations. World Journal of Surgery. 2013;**37**:259-284

[7] Nygren J, Thacker J, Carli F, et al. Guidelines for perioperative care in elective rectal/pelvic surgery: Enhanced recovery after surgery (ERAS(®)) society recommendations. World Journal of Surgery. 2013;**37**:285-305

[8] Gustafsson UO, Scott MJ, Hubner M, et al. Guidelines for perioperative Care in Elective Colorectal Surgery: Enhanced recovery after surgery (ERAS$^{(R)}$) society recommendations: 2018. World Journal of Surgery. 2019;**43**(3):659-695

[9] Gillissen F, Hoff C, Maessen JM, et al. Structured synchronous implementation of an enhanced recovery program in elective colonic surgery in 33 hospitals in the Netherlands. World Journal of Surgery. 2013;**37**:1082-1093

[10] Spanjersberg WR, Reurings J, Keus F, et al. Fast track surgery versus conventional recovery strategies for colorectal surgery. Cochrane Database of Systematic Reviews. 2011;**16**(2):CD007635

[11] Varadhan KK, Lobo DN. A meta-analysis of randomized controlled trials of intravenous fluid therapy in major elective open abdominal surgery: Getting the balance right. The Proceedings of the Nutrition Society. 2010;**69**(4):488-498

[12] Pisarska M, Malczak P, Major P, et al. Enhanced recovery after surgery protocol in oesophageal cancer surgery: Systematic review and meta-analysis. PLoS One. 2017;**12**(3):1-14

[13] De Groot JJA, Ament SMC, Maessen JMC, et al. Enhanced recovery pathways in abdominal gynecologic surgery: A systematic review and meta-analysis. Acta Obstetricia et Gynecologica Scandinavica. 2016;**95**(4):382-395

[14] Ayyadhah AA. Reducing anxiety in preoperative patients: A systematic review. The British Journal of Nursing. 2014;**23**:387-393

[15] Gan TJ, Habib AS, Miller TE, et al. Incidence, patient satisfaction, and perceptions of post-surgical pain: Results from a US national survey. Current Medical Research and Opinion. 2014;**30**:149-160

[16] Hounsome J, Lee A, Greenhalgh J, et al. A systematic review of information format and timing before scheduled adult surgery for peri-operative anxiety. Anaesthesia. 2017;**72**:1265-1272

[17] Wilson CJ, Mitchelson AJ, Tzeng TH, et al. Caring for the surgically anxious patient: A review of the interventions and a guide to optimizing surgical outcomes. American Journal of Surgery. 2016;**212**:151-159

[18] Ziehm S, Rosendahl J, Barth J, et al. Psychological interventions for acute pain after open heart surgery. Cochrane Database of Systematic Reviews. 2017;**7**:CD009984

[19] Dort JC, Farwell DG, Findlay M, et al. Optimal perioperative Care in Major Head and Neck Cancer Surgery with Free Flap Reconstruction: A consensus review and recommendations from the enhanced recovery after surgery society. JAMA Otolaryngology. Head & Neck Surgery. 2017;**143**(3):292-303

[20] Bekelis K, Calnan D, Simmons N, et al. Effect of an immersive preoperative virtual reality experience on patient reported outcomes: A randomized controlled trial. Annals of Surgery. 2017;**265**:1068-1073

[21] Bluman LG, Mosca L, Newman N, et al. Preoperative smoking habits and postoperative pulmonary complications. Chest. 1998;**113**:883-889

[22] Thomsen T, Villebro N, Moller AM. Interventions for preoperative smoking cessation. Cochrane Database of Systematic Reviews. 2014;**2014**(3): CD002294

[23] Mills E, Eyawo O, Lockhart I, et al. Smoking cessation reduces postoperative complications: A systematic review and meta-analysis. The American Journal of Medicine. 2011;**124**(2):144-154

[24] Wong J, Lam DP, Abrishami A, et al. Short-term preoperative smoking cessation and postoperative complications: A systematic review and meta-analysis. Canadian Journal of Anaesthesia. 2012;**59**:268-279

[25] Shabanzadeh DM, Sorensen LT. Alcohol consumption increases post-operative infection but not mortality: A systematic review and meta-analysis. Surgical Infections. 2015;**16**:657-668

[26] Waitzberg DL, Saito H, Plank LD, et al. Postsurgical infections are reduced with specialized nutrition support. World Journal of Surgery. 2006;**30**:1592-1604

[27] American Society of Anesthesiologists Task Force on Perioperative Blood Management. Practice guidelines for perioperative blood management: An updated report by the American Society of Anesthesiologists Task Force on perioperative blood management. Anesthesiology. 2015;**122**:241-275

[28] Gan TJ, Diemunsch P, Habib AS, et al. Consensus guidelines for the management of postoperative nausea and vomiting. Anesthesia and Analgesia. 2014;**118**:85-113

[29] Apfel CC, Kranke P, Eberhart LH, et al. Comparison of predictive models for postoperative nausea and vomiting. British Journal of Anaesthesia. 2002;**88**:234-240

[30] Kappen TH, Moons KG, van Wolfswinkel L, et al. Impact of risk assessments on prophylactic antiemetic prescription and the incidence of postoperative nausea and vomiting: A cluster-randomized trial. Anesthesiology. 2014;**120**:343-354

[31] Kappen TH, Vergouwe Y, van Wolfswinkel L, et al. Impact of adding therapeutic recommendations to risk assessments from a prediction model for postoperative nausea and vomiting. British Journal of Anaesthesia. 2015;**114**:252-260

[32] Ip HY, Abrishami A, Peng PW, et al. Predictors of postoperative pain and analgesic consumption: A qualitative systematic review. Anesthesiology. 2009;**111**:657-677

[33] Tanner J, Norrie P, Melen K. Preoperative hair removal to reduce surgical site infection. Cochrane Database of Systematic Reviews. 2011;**9**(11):CD004122

[34] Practice guidelines for preoperative fasting and the use of pharmacologic agents to reduce the risk of pulmonary aspiration: Application to healthy patients undergoing elective procedures: An updated report by the American Society of Anesthesiologists Task Force on preoperative fasting and the use of pharmacologic agents to reduce the risk of pulmonary aspiration. Anesthesiology. 2017;**126**:376-393

[35] Engelman DT, Ben Ali W, Williams JB, et al. Guidelines for perioperative Care in Cardiac Surgery: Enhanced recovery after surgery society recommendations. JAMA Surgery. 2019;**154**(8):755-766

[36] Medbery RL, Fernandez FG, Khullar OV. ERAS and patient reported outcomes in thoracic surgery: A review of current data. Journal of Thoracic Disease. 2019;**11**(Suppl. 7):S976-S986

[37] Rao W, Zhang X, Zhang J, et al. The role of nasogastric tube in decompression after elective colon and rectum surgery: A meta-analysis. International Journal of Colorectal Disease. 2011;**26**:423-429

[38] Nelson R, Edwards S, Tse B. Prophylactic nasogastric decompression after abdominal surgery. Cochrane Database System. 2007;**2007**(3): CD004929

[39] Kaibori M, Iida H, Ishizaki M, et al. Objective and quantitative assessment of postoperative pain in digestive surgery. In: Kaibori RFM, editor. Enhanced Recovery after Surgery. Singapore: Springer nature; 2018. pp. 29-42

[40] Gregory AJ, Grant MC, Manning MW, et al. Enhanced recovery after cardiac surgery (ERAS cardiac) recommendations: An important first step-but there is much work to Be done. Journal of Cardiothoracic and Vascular Anesthesia. 2020;**34**(1):39-47

[41] Joshi GP, Schug SA, Kehlet H. Procedure-specific pain management and outcome strategies. Best Practice & Research. Clinical Anaesthesiology. 2014;**28**:191-201

[42] Lee B, Schug SA, Joshi GP, et al. Procedure-specific pain management (PROSPECT): An update. Best Practise & Research Anaestheisiology. 2018;**32**:101-111

[43] Hill J, Treasure T. Decreasing the venous thromboembolism risk summary of the NICE guidelines. Praxis (Bern 1994). 2010;**99**:977-980

[44] Kakkos SK, Caprini JA, Geroulakos G, et al. Combined intermittent pneumatic leg compression and pharmacological

prophylaxis for prevention of venous thromboembolism. Cochrane Database of Systematic Reviews. 2016, 2016;**9**:CD005258

[45] Sachdeva A, Dalton M, Lees T. Graduated compression stockings for prevention of deep vein thrombosis. Cochrane Database of Systematic Reviews. 2018;**11**(11):CD001484

[46] Ljungqvist O, Scott M, Fearon KC. Enhanced recovery after surgery: A review. JAMA Surgery. 2017;**152**(3):292-298

[47] Thorell A, Efendic S, Gutniak M, et al. Insulin resistance after abdominal surgery. The British Journal of Surgery. 1994;**81**:59-63

[48] Moningi S, Patki A, Padhy N, et al. Enhanced recovery after surgery: An anesthesiologist's perspective. Journal of Anaesthesiology Clinical Pharmacology. 2019;**35**(Suppl 1):S5-S13

[49] Wisely JC, Barclay KL. Effects of an enhanced recovery after surgery programme on emergency surgical patients. ANZ Journal of Surgery. 2016;**86**(11):883-888

[50] Sharma J, Kumar N, Huda F, et al. Enhanced recovery after surgery protocol in emergency laparotomy: A randomized control study. Surgery Journal (N Y). 2021;**7**(2):e92-e99

[51] Gotlib Conn L, McKenzie M, Pearsall EA, et al. Successful implementation of an enhanced recovery after surgery programme for elective colorectal surgery: A process evaluation of champions' experiences. Implementation Science. 2015;**10**:99

[52] Gustafsson UO, Hausel J, Thorell A. Adherence to the enhanced recovery after surgery protocol and outcomes after colorectal cancer surgery. Archives of Surgery. 2011;**146**:571-577

[53] ERAS Compliance Group. The impact of enhanced recovery protocol compliance on elective colorectal cancer resection: Results from an international registry. Annals of Surgery. 2015;**261**:1153-1159

[54] Glare P, Aubrey KR, Myles PS. Transition from acute to chronic pain after surgery. Lancet. 2019;**393**(10180):1537-1546

[55] Rosero E, Joshi GP. Hospital readmission after ambulatory laparoscopic cholecystectomy: Incidence and predictors. The Journal of Surgical Research. 2017;**219**:108-115

[56] Greco M, Capretti G, Beretta L, et al. Enhanced recovery program in colorectal surgery: A meta-analysis of randomized controlled trials. World Journal of Surgery. 2014;**38**(6):1531-1541

[57] Basse L, Madsen JL, Kehlet H. Normal gastrointestinal transit after colonic resection using epidural analgesia, enforced oral nutrition and laxative. The British Journal of Surgery. 2001;**88**(11):1498-1500

Chapter 4

Pain Management in Enhanced Recovery after Emergency Surgery

K. Madan and Ramya B. Sriram

Abstract

Patients presenting with acute abdominal pain frequently need very good analgesia. In order to obtain successful analgesia, pain should be evaluated, and a suitable intervention should be performed employing multimodal analgesic techniques and a minimum dose of opioid with appropriate monitoring as opioids raise the possibility of the patient being over-sedated, experience hypoventilation, or possibly aspirate. ERAS protocol is a multimodal and multidisciplinary approach to peri-operative management which aims for evidence-based reduction of physiological stress, post-operative complications and organ dysfunction, reoccurrence and mortality whilst also increasing mobility, ultimately leading to early discharge and better surgical outcomes. Multimodal analgesia has an advantage where different techniques are used to tackle pain by targeting different receptors in the pain pathway. Here we discuss a number of multimodal analgesic therapies used to alleviate acute postoperative pain in emergency surgeries, explains their advantages, and evaluates relevant findings and evidence-based management guidelines.

Keywords: postoperative pain, ERAS, emergency surgeries, opioid sparing, multimodal analgesia

1. Introduction

Acute postoperative pain is one of the biggest challenges for both surgeons and anaesthesiologists which affects more than 80% of patients who have surgery with less than 75% of them reporting its severity [1]. However, the use of opioids for pain control in the postoperative period is associated with serious adverse effects like respiratory depression, prolonged hospital stays and opioid addiction on chronic use which impedes enhanced recovery of the patients [2]. Hence enhanced recovery after surgery (ERAS) society has given many guidelines specific to various surgeries which advocates the use of multimodal opioid sparing techniques as they prevent the above-mentioned side effects and helps in early mobilisation and fast return of bowel movements, especially in emergency surgeries [3].

2. Multimodal opioid sparing analgesic techniques

Ideally multimodal analgesia for enhanced recovery should start pre-emptively which prevents central sensitization occurring from incisional and inflammatory injury in the perioperative period. Due to the noxious input brought on by the surgical procedures, the CNS becomes hyperactive, which causes pain hypersensitivity and hyperexcitability (prolonged response of the neurons after tissue damage) which when not treated early may lead to chronic pain. When there is total multi-segmental blockage of unpleasant stimuli and its extension into the postoperative period, the greatest therapeutic improvement is seen. The intensity of immediate postoperative pain/hyperalgesia and chronic pain after surgery might theoretically be decreased or perhaps completely eliminated by preventing central sensitization with comprehensive multimodal analgesic interventions [4, 5].

Multiple strategies and drug classes can be used to control postoperative pain and to allow early mobilisation, enteral nutrition, and to decrease the perioperative stress response. Different techniques like patient education, local anaesthetic-based techniques (local infiltration, peripheral nerve blocks, and neuraxial analgesia), and a combination of analgesic drugs that act via different mechanisms on different receptors can be used [6].

These strategies collectively help in enhanced recovery of the patient and reduces hospital stay.

2.1 Non opioid pharmacological techniques

2.1.1 Acetaminophen

It acts via activating descending serotonergic pathways in the CNS and inhibiting prostaglandin synthesis [7]. When administered intravenously, onset of action is 5 minutes and peak plasma concentrations is attained within 15 minutes [8, 9]. Due to its minimal side effects and varied availability, this drug is widely used in the perioperative period. However, exceeding maximum daily dose of 4 grams in adults and 2–3 grams in frail adults can lead to dose dependant hepatotoxicity and poisoning [10]. When used with NSAIDS, opioid requirement was reduced by 20% [11]. In a study done by Moon et al. with 76 women undergoing abdominal hysterectomy, use of acetaminophen showed reduced requirement of opioid and its associated side effects [12]. Similar results were seen in the RCT study done by Unal et al., in patients undergoing open nephrectomy [13].

2.1.2 Nonsteroidal anti-inflammatory drugs

The mechanism of action is inhibition of cyclooxygenase (COX) and synthesis of prostaglandins, which are mediators of peripheral sensitization and hyperalgesia. The COX1 and COX 2 isoforms act peripherally whereas COX3 isoform acts centrally [14]. COX-1 produces prostaglandins, which are important for general functions such as gastric protection and haemostasis. Whereas COX-2, produces prostaglandins that mediate pain, inflammation, fever, and carcinogenesis.

A systematic review of randomised trials was conducted which showed very clear benefits for selective COX2 inhibitors in reducing postoperative pain and further requirement of analgesia [15]. However, they should not be used in patients with a known history of coronary artery disease or cerebrovascular disease.

NSAIDs significantly decrease opioid-related side effects such as postoperative nausea and vomiting and sedation [16].

The optimal dose of ketorolac (COX1 Inhibitor) for postoperative pain control is 15–30 mg intravenously every 6–8 hours (not to exceed 5 days). However, patients with renal dysfunction should receive a lower dose.

The recommended oral loading dose for Celecoxib (COX-2–specific inhibitor) is a 400 mg followed by 200 mg orally every 12 hours. The dose of injectable COX-2–specific inhibitor parecoxib is 40 mg intravenously or intramuscularly initially followed by 20–40 mg every 4–6 hours not to exceed 80 mg/day.

The nonselective NSAIDs may be avoided during the perioperative phase for a number of reasons, including platelet dysfunction, bronchospasm, gastrointestinal ulcers, and an increased risk of nephrotoxicity especially in patients with hypovolemia, congestive heart failure, and chronic renal insufficiency because prostaglandins dilate the renal vascular beds and mediate diuretic and natriuretic renal effects [17].

Ibuprofen IV and intranasal ketorolac are two newer NSAID formulations that have been approved for the treatment of immediate postoperative pain.

A meta-analysis done by Martinez et al. showed efficacy best with α-2 agonists, NSAIDs and COX-2 inhibitors when used alone and least with tramadol and acetaminophen [18].

In order to avoid systemic side effects transdermal patches can be used which have proven as efficacious as other routes of administration. In the study done by Bhargava et al., it is seen that diclofenac sodium patch proved to be as effective as diclofenac sodium intramuscular injection in post operative analgesia. With added advantages of longer onset of action, lesser local side effects like skin erythema, pruritis, oedema, abscess and necrosis and lesser gastrointestinal effects [19].

2.1.3 N-methyl D Aspartate (NMDA) Receptor Antagonists

The spinal cord N-methyl-D-aspartate (NMDA) receptors are activated by glutamate when C-fibre nociceptors fire repeatedly. Central sensitization results from the activation of NMDA receptors, which makes spinal cord neurons more receptive to all of their inputs thus causing prolonged postoperative pain.

Ketamine acts by non-competitively inhibiting NMDA receptors [20]. It also interacts with opioid, cholinergic, and monoaminergic receptors and blocks sodium channels [21]. Ketamine reduces postoperative pain significantly and also reduces opioid tolerance [22] and rescue analgesic requirements and pain intensity [23]. In a systematic review, it was discovered that IV ketamine for postoperative analgesia was an efficient adjunct, especially in patients undergoing major upper abdominal, thoracic, and orthopaedic surgeries [24]. Low-dose ketamine (0.25–0.5 mg intravenous bolus followed by an infusion of 2–4 μg/kg/min) can provide significant analgesia and is opioid-sparing.

Major side effect of ketamine is its impact on cognitive level (such as hallucinations, vivid dreams, diplopia, blurred vision, nystagmus, or dysphoria) of the patient which is usually not seen when administered in analgesic doses [25].

Dextromethorphan also acts by non-competitively inhibiting NMDA receptors. However, it poses a variety of side effects like nausea and vomiting (oral preparation) and hypotension and tachycardia (on large intravenous does). Hence intramuscular route od administration is preferred.

Magnesium also acts by non-competitively inhibiting NMDA receptors. A study done by Albrecht et al. showed that when magnesium was given intravenously peri-operatively, it could reduce opioid consumption, and also pain scores, in the first 24 hrs postoperatively, without any serious adverse effects [26]. Two different meta-analysis showed that magnesium showed reduction of pain both at rest and on movement with reduced postoperative requirement of opioids [27, 28].

2.1.4 Gabapentinoids

These were earlier developed as anti-epileptic drugs for the treatment of partial onset seizures which was later found to have analgesic properties and hence was used in neuropathic pain (e.g., postherpetic neuralgia), and other chronic pain states (e.g., fibromyalgia). These drugs have been recently used for acute perioperative pain relief also. These opioid sparing analgesics also have added advantage of reduced incidence of postoperative vomiting, pruritus, and urinary retention.

Tissue damage makes dorsal horn neurons hyperexcited which is decreased by gabapentinoids. They bind presynaptically with calcium receptors (both in central and peripheral nervous system) thus redistributing the calcium channels away from its functional membrane bound site to its non-functional cytosolic site [29, 30].

The dose given to manage postoperative pain in an adult is 900 mg of gabapentin orally, 1–2 hours before surgery [31]. A saturable transport system in the gastrointestinal tract allows for the absorption of gabapentin, which results in a decline in bioavailability with increasing doses. As a result, as the drug dose is raised, the plasma drug concentration grows gradually less (e.g., nonlinear pharmacokinetics [32].

Pregabalin has better potency and lesser side effects compared to gabapentin for the treating of acute perioperative pain. A RCT study showed that when pregabalin was given at a dose of 150 mg twice daily, it reduced preoperative anxiety and postoperative pain scores and analgesic requirement with better sleep quality [33]. A study done by Bekawi et al. showed that pregabalin when given perioperatively per orally with a dose of 150 mg, it proved to be very effective for postoperative pain when compared to pethidine [34].

2.1.5 Intravenous lidocaine

Lidocaine, an amide local anaesthetic and class 1b antiarrhythmic, when given intravenously inhibits voltage-gated sodium channels, voltage-gated calcium channels, various potassium channels, NMDA receptors, glycine system, and G protein pathways [35] and thus prevents hypersensitization and hyperalgesia [36].

Numerous clinical investigations indicate that perioperative systemic lidocaine administration reduces the release of pro-inflammatory cytokines caused by surgical stress [37–39].

Some studies showed that when lidocaine infusion with dose 2 mg/kg/hr. was given intraoperatively and postoperatively for 8 hrs in patients undergoing laparotomy or laparoscopic abdominal surgery, there was quicker return of bowel movements and reduced postoperative pain, hence reduced need of opioid consumption [40–42].

However, some studies have reported a few adverse drug reactions associated with systemic lidocaine administration like drowsiness, perioral numbness, nausea and blood pressure changes [43]. Systemic lidocaine showed be used cautiously in patients with cardiac arrhythmias.

Lidocaine is also available as transdermal patches which when applied on the laparoscopic port sites reduced postoperative pain [44].

2.1.6 Alpha-2 agonists

Analgesia is primarily mediated by presynaptic stimulation of alpha 2-receptors, which causes a reduction in the release of norepinephrine. Analgesia works at 3 sites, supraspinally (locus coeruleus), spinally (substantia gelatinosa), and peripherally.

Both clonidine and dexmedetomidine are selective partial agonists for the α2-adrenoreceptor, but the latter is 8 times more selective than the former.

Analgesia is seen supraspinally (locus coeruleus), spinally (substantia gelatinosa), and peripherally [45].

Dexmedetomidine has advantages over clonidine analgesia, titratable sedation (e.g., "cooperative sedation"), anxiolysis, cardioprotective, prevent respiratory depression associated with ketamine and opioid [46]. Loading dose of dexmedetomidine is 1 μg/kg intravenous over 10 minutes and maintenance dose is infusion of 0.2–0.7 μg/kg/hr [47].

2.1.7 Glucocorticoids

Analgesic effect mainly occurs due to by inhibiting leukotriene and prostaglandin production.

A recent study done by Koc et al. showed that when dexamethasone (8 mg intravenously) and gabapentin (800 mg orally) were administered together 1 hour prior to varicocele surgery, postoperative analgesia was much better [48].

2.1.8 Surgical site infiltration

Intraperitoneal local anaesthetics- Here the local anaesthetic is sprayed in the right subdiaphragmatic region in patients undergoing laparoscopic cholecystectomy at the beginning of the procedure. Many trials have shown significant positive results proving its efficacy extending to postoperative period. Local anaesthetics like lidocaine or bupivacaine can be used in different concentrations and volume [49, 50]. It has also been efficacious in other laparoscopic surgeries like gynaecological laparoscopy, sterilisation, fundoplication, appendectomy, etc. with postoperative analgesia upto 24 hours and reduced analgesia consumption by 50% [51].

Trocar and port site infiltration with local anaesthetics- Many studies have shown that trocar and port site infiltration of local anaesthetic in various layers of the abdominal wall is very helpful like in the preperitoneal or subfascial or subcutaneous layers [52–54]. A study done by Candiotti et al., used opioid-based intravenous patient-controlled analgesia (PCA) and liposome bupivacaine in patients undergoing laparoscopic colectomy. Here long-acting liposomal formulation of bupivacaine is infiltrated in the surgical site. This technique proved to show lower requirement of opioid and shorter duration of hospital stay [55].

2.2 Preoperative patient pain education and preparedness

Literature shows that postoperative pain remains undertreated despite decades of education and evidence-based guidelines [56]. Counselling and educating the patient and their family both preoperatively and postoperatively regarding the pain and its management plays a pivotal role in reduced pharmacological means of analgesia, especially opioids and sedatives [57].

2.3 Neuraxial analgesic techniques

Epidural analgesia is a key component of multimodal analgesia which can either be given as single shot dose or continuously with a catheter placed in situ. Successful epidural analgesia depends on a number of factors like site of catheter insertion, choice of analgesic drugs, rates of infusion, duration of analgesia, and type of pain (rest or dynamic).

Epidural analgesia works by, spinal and supraspinal mechanism. Spinal mechanism occurs when the drug diffuses into cerebrospinal fluid.

Better analgesia is seen when a local anaesthetic is combined with an opioid for epidural analgesia because when given epidurally opioid is devoid of significant sympatholytic and motor blockade and also the combination has synergistic effect. Adjuncts like clonidine and ketamine can also be added to improve duration and efficacy.

Epidural analgesia is contraindicated in a few conditions like severe coagulation abnormalities like disseminated intravascular coagulation. Cautious use in case of sepsis, increased intracranial pressure, thrombocytopenia, pre-existing central nervous system disorder, previous back surgery, pre-existing neurologic injury, back pain, etc.

Extended-release epidural morphine was also found effective for lower abdominal surgeries where the opioid, morphine in in a liposome delivery system. This system controls the release of morphine over a period of 48 hours postoperatively [58].

Intrathecal analgesia is a also widely accepted especially with opioids [59]. Other adjuncts can also be used like α2-agonists, NSAIDs, NMDA receptor antagonists, acetylcholinesterase inhibitors, adenosine, epinephrine, and benzodiazepines.

2.4 Peripheral nerve blocks

There are numerous peripheral nerve blocks that enhance analgesia for both intraoperative and postoperative pain due to abdominal surgeries (both laparoscopic and laparotomy). These blocks can either be performed under landmark technique or ultrasound guided. Some of the blocks that will be discussed in brief with respect to abdominal surgeries are transversus abdominis plane (TAP) block, paravertebral block, rectus sheath block, quadratus lumborum block, ilioinguinal and iliohypogastric block, erector spinae and other interfascial blocks.

2.4.1 Transversus abdominis plane (TAP) block

Four major muscles are considered with respect to transversus abdominis plane (TAP) block. The transversus abdominis plane contains T6–L1 thoracolumbar nerves which supply sensitivity to the skin and muscles of the anterior abdominal wall, upper hip, groin, and thigh.

The landmark technique block is performed at the level of the Petit triangle (formed by the iliac crest as the inferior border, the latissimus dorsi as the posterior border, and the external oblique as the anterior border) with patient in supine position. The local anaesthetic is deposited when 2 pops are felt while advancing the needle in the triangle of petit.

There are various approaches to ultrasound guided TAP block like subcostal, lateral and posterior approaches.

A meta-analysis done by Yu n et al. showed that 24 hours VAS score in patients with TAP block was much less compared to patients who were given local wound infiltration [60]. A meta-analysis done by Zhao et al. showed that TAP block used in laparoscopic surgeries reduced the analgesic requirement postoperatively [61].

2.4.2 Rectus abdominus block

Rectus sheath is formed mainly by the aponeurosis of 3 main abdominal wall muscles (external oblique, internal oblique and the transversus abdominis muscles) which thus surrounds the rectus abdominus muscle. This sheath contains nerves from ventral rami arising from T7 to T11 intercostal nerves and the subcostal nerve (T12). This block is mainly useful in umbilical surgeries. This block is best performed under ultrasound guidance. With the transducer placed in the midline at the level of the umbilicus, the needle is passed through the rectus abdomnus muscle till the tip is on the posterior rectus sheath. Where the local anaesthetic is deposited.

In the study done by Kartaloy et al., the results showed that the patients who received rectus abdominus muscle block for abdominal surgeries requiring general anaesthesia had lower pain scores and reduced need for morphine when compared to patients who were given general anaesthesia alone [62].

In a study done by Gunaney et al., ultrasound guided rectus abdominus block was better than surgical site infiltration of local anaesthetic in patients undergoing umbilical hernia surgeries [63].

2.4.3 Ilioinguinal/iliohypogastric nerve block

Both these nerves arise from L1 supplies sensory inputs to the skin of the lower abdominal wall, upper hip and upper thigh. This block has shown good analgesia in inguinal hernia surgeries especially in children.

In a study done on cadavers showed 95% successful block rates done under ultrasound guidance compared to blind technique [64].

A study done by Demirci et al. showed that this block done under ultrasound guidance for adult herniorrhaphies is better than landmark technique for providing postoperative analgesia [65].

2.4.4 Thoracic paravertebral block

This block is mainly useful for breast and thoracic surgeries but can also be used for upper abdominal surgeries when given at the level T6–T12 for providing postoperative analgesia.

Studies were done where sole thoracic paravertebral block was compared to spinal anaesthesia for inguinal hernia surgeries which showed lower pain scores in the early postoperative period [66–69].

A study was done by Kaya et al. comparing the efficacy of thoracic paravertebral block and transversus abdominis plane block as adjunct where the former proved to be better as postoperative analgesia. This block has given good results also for cholecystectomy (both open and laparoscopic) [70–72] and ventral hernia surgeries and other urological and gynaecological procedures.

2.4.5 Erector spinae plane (ESP) block

It is an inter-fascial plane, where the local anaesthetic when deposited affects both the ventral and dorsal branches of the thoracic spinal nerves and the rami communicants that contain sympathetic nerve fibres. When given for abdominal surgeries at the level of T7, it gives both visceral and somatic analgesia. When administered the local anaesthetic spreads in both cranial and caudal directions [73, 74].

A study done by Altıparmak et al., showed erector spinae plane (US-ESP) block given under ultrasound guidance reduced the opioid requirement and pain scores postoperatively compared to TAP block for laparoscopic cholecystectomy cases [75].

2.4.6 Quadratus lumborum (QL) block

It is an interfascial block where the local anaesthetic is administered in thoracolumbar fascia which encloses quadratus lumborum, psoas major, and the erector spinae muscles which extends from T6-L1 [76].

This local anaesthetic provides blockade to referred dermatome.

Many case reports are published proving its efficacy for postoperative analgesia in major laparotomies. Two case reports done by Kadam et al. showed that QL block when given for open right hemi colectomy with a midline incision and laparotomy for duodenal tumour excision as a component of multimodal analgesia showed significant reduction of dynamic pain scores in the subsequent postoperative period [77, 78].

Another case report was done for a patient undergoing subtotal colectomy for ulcerative colitis where the patient received transmuscular QL block on the left side and TAP block on the right side (right side as control). It was found that sensation on the left side from T8-L1 was reduced and persisted for 48 hours while on the right side the sensation reduced from T10-L1 which only lasted for 48 hours.

2.5 Cognitive behavioural therapies (CBT)

Along with pharmaceutical medications, it can be employed as a component of multimodal pain control during the healing process (weak recommendation). The stress associated with anxiety for surgery aggravates pain and this will become a vicious cycle. Hence different types of cognitive behavioural therapies act like adjuncts in alleviating pain. The various types of cognitive behavioural therapies are music therapy, relaxation techniques, guided imagery, intraoperative conversation with patient, hypnosis, electro analgesia in the form of transcutaneous or peripheral electrical nerve stimulation and acupuncture [79–81].

Music therapy alleviates pain by attention shift or cognitive coping [82]. Role of music in the postoperative period was studied by Hole et al. in the form of a systematic review. It was seen that patients who used music with noise cancelling headphones during trans rectal biopsy were found to have lesser pain scores compared to use of noise-cancelling headphones alone [83]. Another analysis done with 73 randomised controlled studies and 20,458 patients showed that music reduced both post-operative pain and anxiety and hence increased patient satisfaction scores. Music therapy was also seen to be beneficial when patients were under general anaesthesia [84]. However, more research is necessary for establishing evidence on the type and duration of music therapy for adequate opioid sparing.

A randomised control trial done in patients undergoing breast cancer surgeries showed the reduced requirement of propofol and lidocaine when these patients underwent clinical hypnosis [85].

3. Conclusion

Good perioperative pain control is the key for early recovery in enhanced recovery after surgery (ERAS) especially in emergency surgeries. It is important for the clinicians to have patient-oriented strategies for the overall faster recovery of these patients. It is crucial to begin pain relief therapy before the surgery because patients scheduled for emergency surgeries already endure excruciating pain. Hence for early recovery opioid sparing multimodal analgesia management should be followed as advocated by ERAS. Use of multiple modalities in treating perioperative pain helps reduce the dose and side effects of a single drug or modality. This strategy has been demonstrated to enhance prospects for these patients with very high risks. Use of regional anaesthetic procedures should be promoted as improved results are observed. The goal here should be to provide appropriate and safer pain management methods to reduce perioperative pain.

Conflict of interest

The authors declare no conflict of interest.

Author details

K. Madan[1] and Ramya B. Sriram[2]*

1 Department of Surgery, Ramaiah Medical College, Bangalore, India

2 Department of Anesthesiology and Critical Care, Bangalore Medical College and Research Institute, Bangalore, India

*Address all correspondence to: ramyabsriram6@gmail.com

References

[1] Chou R, Gordon DB, de Leon-Casasola OA, Rosenberg JM, Bickler S, Brennan T, et al. Management of Postoperative Pain: A clinical practice guideline from the American pain society, the American Society of Regional Anesthesia and Pain Medicine, and the American Society of Anesthesiologists' committee on regional Anesthesia, executive committee, and administrative council. The Journal of Pain. 2016;**17**(2):131-157

[2] Dahan A, Aarts L, Smith TW. Incidence, reversal, and prevention of opioid-induced respiratory depression. Anesthesiology. 2010;**112**(1):226-238

[3] Peden CJ, Aggarwal G, Aitken RJ, Anderson ID, Bang Foss N, Cooper Z, et al. Guidelines for perioperative Care for Emergency Laparotomy Enhanced Recovery after Surgery (ERAS) society recommendations: Part 1—Preoperative: Diagnosis, rapid assessment and optimization. World Journal of Surgery. 2021;**45**(5):1272-1290

[4] Møiniche S, Kehlet H, Dahl JB. A qualitative and quantitative systematic review of Preemptive analgesia for postoperative pain relief. Anesthesiology. 2002;**96**(3):725-741

[5] Perkins FM, Kehlet H. Chronic pain as an outcome of surgery. Anesthesiology. 2000;**93**(4):1123-1133

[6] Kehlet H, Holte K. Effect of postoperative analgesia on surgical outcome. British Journal of Anaesthesia. 2001;**87**(1):62-72

[7] Sinatra RS, Jahr JS, Reynolds L, Groudine SB, Royal MA, Breitmeyer JB, et al. Intravenous acetaminophen for pain after major Orthopedic surgery: An expanded analysis: IV acetaminophen for pain after major Orthopedic surgery. Pain Practice. 2012;**12**(5):357-365

[8] McNicol ED, Ferguson MC, Haroutounian S, Carr DB, Schumann R. Single dose intravenous paracetamol or intravenous propacetamol for postoperative pain. Cochrane Pain, Palliative and Supportive Care Group. Cochrane Database System Review. 2016;**2016**:23. DOI: 10.1002/14651858.CD007126.pub3

[9] Liukas A, Kuusniemi K, Aantaa R, Virolainen P, Niemi M, Neuvonen PJ, et al. Pharmacokinetics of intravenous paracetamol in elderly patients. Clinical Pharmacokinetics. 2011;**50**(2):121-129

[10] American Geriatrics Society Panel on the Pharmacological Management of Persistent Pain in Older Persons. Pharmacological Management of Persistent Pain in Older Persons: Pharmacological management of persistent pain in older persons. Journal of American Geriatric Society. 2009;**57**(8):1331-1346

[11] Cao X, Elvir-Lazo OL, White PF, Yumul R, Tang J. An update on pain management for elderly patients undergoing ambulatory surgery. Current Opinion in Anaesthesiology. 2016;**29**(6):674-682

[12] Moon YE, Lee YK, Lee J, Moon DE. The effects of preoperative intravenous acetaminophen in patients undergoing abdominal hysterectomy. Archives of Gynecology and Obstetrics. 2011;**284**(6):1455-1460

[13] Unal SS, Aksoy M, Ahiskalioglu A, Erdem AF, Adanur S. The effect of intravenous preemptive paracetamol on

postoperative fentanyl consumption in patients undergoing open nephrectomy: A prospective randomized study. Nigerian Journal of Clinical Practice. 2015;**18**(1):68-74

[14] Svensson CI, Yaksh TL. The spinal phospholipase-cyclooxygenase-Prostanoid Cascade in nociceptive processing. Annual Review of Pharmacology and Toxicology. 2002;**42**(1):553-583

[15] Straube S, Derry S, McQuay HJ, Moore RA. Effect of preoperative Cox-II-selective NSAIDs (coxibs) on postoperative outcomes: A systematic review of randomized studies. Acta Anaesthesiologica Scandinavica. 2005;**49**(5):601-613

[16] Marret E, Kurdi O, Zufferey P, Bonnet F, Warltier DC. Effects of nonsteroidal Antiinflammatory drugs on patient-controlled analgesia morphine side effects. Anesthesiology. 2005;**102**(6):1249-1260

[17] Rowlingson JC, Eisenach JC. Essentials of pain medicine and regional Anesthesia. Anesthesiology. 2001;**94**(6):1154-1154

[18] Martinez V, Beloeil H, Marret E, Fletcher D, Ravaud P, Trinquart L. Non-opioid analgesics in adults after major surgery: Systematic review with network meta-analysis of randomized trials. British Journal of Anaesthesia. 2017;**118**(1):22-31

[19] Bhargava G, Bansal D, Sidhu A, Bhatia A. Diclofenac patch: A better alternative to injectable diclofenac in postoperative pain management. International Surgery Journal. Nov 2015;**2**(4):623-628

[20] Thomson AM, West DC, Lodge D. An N-methylaspartate receptor-mediated synapse in rat cerebral cortex: A site of action of ketamine? Nature. 1985;**313**(6002):479-481

[21] Weinbroum AA. A single small dose of postoperative ketamine provides rapid and sustained improvement in morphine analgesia in the presence of morphine-resistant pain. Anesthesia and Analgesia. 2003;**2003**:789-795

[22] Laskowski K, Stirling A, McKay WP, Lim HJ. A systematic review of intravenous ketamine for postoperative analgesia. Canadian Journal of Anesthesia. 2011;**58**(10):911-923

[23] Dahmani S, Michelet D, Abback PS, Wood C, Brasher C, Nivoche Y, et al. Ketamine for perioperative pain management in children: A meta-analysis of published studies: Ketamine for perioperative analgesia. Pediatric Anesthesia. 2011;**21**(6):636-652

[24] Morgan CJA, Curran HV. Acute and chronic effects of ketamine upon human memory: A review. Psychopharmacology. 2006;**188**(4):408-424

[25] Altunkaya H, Ozer Y, Kargi E, Ozkocak I, Hosnuter M, Demirel CB, et al. The postoperative analgesic effect of tramadol when used as subcutaneous local anesthetic. Anaesthesia Analgesic. Nov 2004;**99**(5):1461-1464

[26] Albrecht E, Kirkham KR, Liu SS, Brull R. Peri-operative intravenous administration of magnesium sulphate and postoperative pain: A meta-analysis: Peri-operative intravenous magnesium and postoperative pain. Anaesthesia. 2013;**68**(1):79-90

[27] De Oliveira GS, Castro-Alves LJ, Khan JH, McCarthy RJ. Perioperative systemic magnesium to minimize postoperative pain. Anesthesiology. 2013;**119**(1):178-190

[28] Murphy JD, Paskaradevan J, Eisler LL, Ouanes JPP, Tomas VAG, Freck EA, et al. Analgesic efficacy of continuous intravenous magnesium infusion as an adjuvant to morphine for postoperative analgesia: A systematic review and meta-analysis. Middle East Journal of Anaesthesiology. 2013;**22**(1):11-20

[29] Zhang J, Ho KY, Wang Y. Efficacy of pregabalin in acute postoperative pain: A meta-analysis. British Journal of Anaesthesia. 2011;**106**(4):454-462

[30] Taylor CP. Mechanisms of analgesia by gabapentin and pregabalin—Calcium channel α2-δ [Cavα2-δ] ligands. Pain. 2009;**142**(1):13-16

[31] Turan A, White PF, Karamanlioğlu B, Memis D, Taşdoğan M, Pamukçu Z, et al. Gabapentin: An alternative to the Cyclooxygenase-2 inhibitors for perioperative pain management. Anesthesia and Analgesia. 2006;**102**(1):175-181

[32] Gilron I. Gabapentin and pregabalin for chronic neuropathic and early postsurgical pain: Current evidence and future directions. Current Opinion in Anaesthesiology. 2007;**20**(5):456-472

[33] Shimony N, Amit U, Minz B, Grossman R, Dany MA, Gonen L, et al. Perioperative pregabalin for reducing pain, analgesic consumption, and anxiety and enhancing sleep quality in elective neurosurgical patients: A prospective, randomized, double-blind, and controlled clinical study. Journal of Neurosurgery. 2016;**125**(6):1513-1522

[34] Bekawi MS, El Wakeel LM, Al Taher WMA, Mageed WMA. Clinical study evaluating Pregabalin efficacy and tolerability for pain Management in Patients Undergoing Laparoscopic Cholecystectomy. The Clinical Journal of Pain. 2014;**30**(11):944-952

[35] van der Wal SEI, van den Heuvel SAS, Radema SA, van Berkum BFM, Vaneker M, Steegers MAH, et al. The *in vitro* mechanisms and *in vivo* efficacy of intravenous lidocaine on the neuroinflammatory response in acute and chronic pain. European Journal of Pain. 2016;**20**(5):655-674

[36] Kawamata M, Takahashi T, Kozuka Y, Nawa Y, Nishikawa K, Narimatsu E, et al. Experimental incision-induced pain in human skin: Effects of systemic lidocaine on flare formation and hyperalgesia. Pain. 2002;**100**(1):77-89

[37] Kuo CP, Jao SW, Chen KM, Wong CS, Yeh CC, Sheen MJ, et al. Comparison of the effects of thoracic epidural analgesia and i.v. infusion with lidocaine on cytokine response, postoperative pain and bowel function in patients undergoing colonic surgery. British Journal of Anaesthesia. 2006;**97**(5):640-646

[38] Yardeni IZ, Beilin B, Mayburd E, Levinson Y, Bessler H. The effect of perioperative intravenous lidocaine on postoperative pain and immune function. Anesthesia and Analgesia. 2009;**109**(5):1464-1469

[39] Sridhar P, Sistla SC, Ali SM, Karthikeyan VS, Badhe AS, Ananthanarayanan PH. Effect of intravenous lignocaine on perioperative stress response and post-surgical ileus in elective open abdominal surgeries: A double-blind randomized controlled trial: Attenuation of stress response with lignocaine. ANZ Journal of Surgery. 2015;**85**(6):425-429

[40] Sun Y, Li T, Wang N, Yun Y, Gan TJ. Perioperative systemic lidocaine for postoperative analgesia and recovery after abdominal surgery: A Meta-analysis of randomized controlled trials. Diseases of the Colon and Rectum. 2012;**55**(11):1183-1194

[41] McCarthy GC, Megalla SA, Habib AS. Impact of intravenous lidocaine infusion on postoperative analgesia and recovery from surgery: A systematic review of randomized controlled trials. Drugs. 2010;**70**(9):1149-1163

[42] Dunn LK, Durieux ME. Perioperative use of intravenous lidocaine. Anesthesiology. 2017;**126**(4):729-737

[43] Peixoto RD, Hawley P. Intravenous lidocaine for Cancer pain without electrocardiographic monitoring: A retrospective review. Journal of Palliative Medicine. 2015;**18**(4):373-377

[44] Kwon YS, Kim JB, Jung HJ, Koo YJ, Lee IH, Im KT, et al. Treatment for postoperative wound pain in Gynecologic laparoscopic surgery: Topical lidocaine patches. Journal of Laparoendoscopic Advances Surgery Technology. 2012;**22**(7):668-673

[45] Chan AKM, Cheung CW, Chong YK. Alpha-2 agonists in acute pain management. Expert Opinion on Pharmacotherapy. 2010;**11**(17):2849-2868

[46] Ebert T, Maze M. Dexmedetomidine: Another arrow for the Clinician's quiver. Anesthesiology. 2004;**101**(3):568-570

[47] Gerlach AT, Dasta JF. Dexmedetomidine: An updated review. The Annals of Pharmacotherapy. 2007;**41**(2):245-254

[48] Koç S, Memis D, Sut N. The preoperative use of gabapentin, dexamethasone, and their combination in Varicocele surgery: A randomized controlled trial. Anesthesia and Analgesia. 2007;**105**(4):1137-1142

[49] Weber A, Muñoz J, Garteiz D, Cueto J. Use of subdiaphragmatic bupivacaine instillation to control postoperative pain after laparoscopic surgery. Surgical Laparoscopy & Endoscopy. 1997;**7**(1):6-8

[50] Mraovič B, Jurišič T, Kogler-Majeric V, Sustic A. Intraperitoneal bupivacaine for analgesia after laparoscopic cholecystectomy. Acta Anaesthesiologica Scandinavica. 1997;**41**(2):193-196

[51] Cunniffe MG, McAnena OJ, Dar MA, Calleary J, Flynn N. A prospective randomized trial of intraoperative bupivacaine irrigation for management of shoulder-tip pain following laparoscopy. American Journal of Surgery. 1998;**176**(3):258-261

[52] Ke R. A randomized, double-blinded trial of preemptive analgesia in laparoscopy. Obstetrics and Gynecology. 1998;**92**(6):972-975

[53] Saff GN, Marks RA, Kuroda M, Rozan JP, Hertz R. Analgesic effect of bupivacaine on extraperitoneal laparoscopic hernia repair. Anesthesia Analgesia. 1998;**87**(2):377-381

[54] Deans GT, Wilson MS, Brough WA. Controlled trial of preperitoneal local anaesthetic for reducing pain following laparoscopic hernia repair. The British Journal of Surgery. 2003;**85**(7):1013-1014

[55] Candiotti KA, Sands LR, Lee E, Bergese SD, Harzman AE, Marcet J, et al. Liposome bupivacaine for postsurgical analgesia in adult patients undergoing laparoscopic colectomy: Results from prospective phase IV sequential cohort studies assessing health economic outcomes. Current Therapeutic Research. 2014;**76**:1-6

[56] O'Donnell KF. Preoperative pain management education: A quality improvement project. Journal of Perianesthesia Nursing. 2015;**30**(3):221-227

[57] Khorfan R, Shallcross ML, Yu B, Sanchez N, Parilla S, Coughlin JM, et al.

Preoperative patient education and patient preparedness are associated with less postoperative use of opioids. Surgery. 2020;**167**(5):852-858

[58] Hartrick CT, Hartrick KA. Extended-release epidural morphine (DepoDur™): Review and safety analysis. Expert Review of Neurotherapeutics. 2008;**8**(11):1641-1648

[59] Rathmell JP, Lair TR, Nauman B. The role of intrathecal drugs in the treatment of acute pain. Anesthesia and Analgesia. 2005;**101**(5S):S30-S43

[60] Yu N, Long X, Lujan-Hernandez JR, Succar J, Xin X, Wang X. Transversus abdominis-plane block versus local anesthetic wound infiltration in lower abdominal surgery: A systematic review and meta-analysis of randomized controlled trials. BMC Anesthesiology. 2014;**14**(1):121

[61] Zhao X, Tong Y, Ren H, Ding XB, Wang X, Zong JY, et al. Transversus abdominis plane block for postoperative analgesia after laparoscopic surgery: A systematic review and meta-analysis. International Journal of Clinical and Experimental Medicine. 2014;7(9):2966-2975

[62] Kartalov A, Jankulovski N, Kuzmanovska B, Zdravkovska M, Shosholcheva M, Tolevska M, et al. The effect of rectus sheath block as a supplement of general Anesthesia on postoperative analgesia in adult patient undergoing umbilical hernia repair. Prilozi. 2017;**38**(3):135-142

[63] Gurnaney HG, Maxwell LG, Kraemer FW, Goebel T, Nance ML, Ganesh A. Prospective randomized observer-blinded study comparing the analgesic efficacy of ultrasound-guided rectus sheath block and local anaesthetic infiltration for umbilical hernia repair. British Journal of Anaesthesia. 2011;**107**(5):790-795

[64] Eichenberger U, Greher M, Kirchmair L, Curatolo M, Moriggl B. Ultrasound-guided blocks of the ilioinguinal and iliohypogastric nerve: Accuracy of a selective new technique confirmed by anatomical dissection. British Journal of Anaesthesia. 2006;**97**(2):238-243

[65] Demirci A, Efe EM, Türker G, Gurbet A, Kaya FN, Anil A, et al. Iliohypogastric/ilioinguinal nerve block in inguinal hernia repair for postoperative pain management: Comparison of the anatomical landmark and ultrasound guided techniques. Revista Brasileira de Anestesiologia. 2014;**64**(5):350-356

[66] Akcaboy EY, Akcaboy ZN, Gogus N. Ambulatory inguinal herniorrhaphy: Paravertebral block versus spinal anesthesia. Minerva Anestesiologica. 2009;**75**(12):684-691

[67] Bhattacharya P, Mandal MC, Mukhopadhyay S, Das S, Pal PP, Basu SR. Unilateral paravertebral block: An alternative to conventional spinal anaesthesia for inguinal hernia repair. Acta Anaesthesiologica Scandinavica. 2010;**54**(2):246-251

[68] Mandal MC, Das S, Gupta S, Ghosh TR, Basu SR. Paravertebral block can be an alternative to unilateral spinal anaesthesia for inguinal hernia repair. Indian Journal of Anaesthesia. 2011;**55**(6):584-589

[69] Fusco P, Cofini V, Petrucci E, Scimia P, Paladini G, Behr AU, et al. Unilateral paravertebral block compared with subarachnoid anesthesia for the management of postoperative pain syndrome after inguinal herniorrhaphy: A randomized controlled clinical trial. Pain. 2016;**157**(5):1105-1113

[70] Agarwal A, Batra RK, Chhabra A, Subramaniam R, Misra MC. The evaluation of efficacy and safety of paravertebral block for perioperative analgesia in patients undergoing laparoscopic cholecystectomy. Saudi Journal of Anaesthesia. 2012;**6**(4):344-349

[71] Abou Zeid HA, Al-Ghamdi AMA, Abdel-Hadi MSA, Zakaria HM, Al-Quorain AAA, Shawkey MN. Bilateral paravertebral block in advanced schistosomal liver disease: A prospective study. Saudi Journal of Gastroenterological Official Journal of Saudi Gastroenterological Association. 2004;**10**(2):67-77

[72] Naja MZ, Ziade MF, Lönnqvist PA. General anaesthesia combined with bilateral paravertebral blockade (T5-6) vs. general anaesthesia for laparoscopic cholecystectomy: A prospective, randomized clinical trial. European Journal of Anaesthesiology. 2004;**21**(6):489-495

[73] Chin KJ, Adhikary S, Sarwani N, Forero M. The analgesic efficacy of pre-operative bilateral erector spinae plane (ESP) blocks in patients having ventral hernia repair. Anaesthesia. 2017;**72**(4):452-460

[74] Restrepo-Garces CE, Chin KJ, Suarez P, Diaz A. Bilateral continuous erector Spinae plane block contributes to effective postoperative analgesia after major open abdominal surgery: A case report. Case Report. 2017;**9**(11):319-321

[75] Altıparmak B, Korkmaz Toker M, Uysal AI, Kuşçu Y, Gümüş DS. Ultrasound-guided erector spinae plane block versus oblique subcostal transversus abdominis plane block for postoperative analgesia of adult patients undergoing laparoscopic cholecystectomy: Randomized, controlled trial. Journal of Clinical Anesthesia. 2019;**57**:31-36

[76] Visoiu M, Yakovleva N. Continuous postoperative analgesia via quadratus lumborum block—An alternative to transversus abdominis plane block. Pediatric Anesthesia. 2013;**23**(10):959-961

[77] Kadam V. Ultrasound-guided quadratus lumborum block as a postoperative analgesic technique for laparotomy. Journal of Anaesthesiology Clinical Pharmacology. 2013;**29**(4):550

[78] Kadam V. Ultrasound guided quadratus lumborum block or posterior transversus abdominis plane block catheter infusion as a postoperative analgesic technique for abdominal surgery. Journal of Anaesthesiology Clinical Pharmacology. 2015;**31**(1):130

[79] Zhang Q, Li YN, Guo YY, Yin CP, Gao F, Xin X, et al. Effects of preconditioning of electro-acupuncture on postoperative cognitive dysfunction in elderly: A prospective, randomized, controlled trial. Medicine (Baltimore). 2017;**96**(26):e7375

[80] Meissner W. The role of acupuncture and transcutaneous-electrical nerve stimulation for postoperative pain control. Current Opinion in Anaesthesiology. 2009;**22**(5):623-626

[81] Chandra A, Banavaliker J, Das P, Hasti S. Use of transcutaneous electrical nerve stimulation as an adjunctive to epidural analgesia in the management of acute thoracotomy pain. Indian Journal of Anaesthesia. 2010;**54**(2):116

[82] Pyati S, Gan TJ. Perioperative pain management. CNS Drugs. 2007;**21**(3):185-211

[83] Tsivian M, Qi P, Kimura M, Chen VH, Chen SH, Gan TJ, et al. The effect of noise-cancelling headphones or music on pain perception and anxiety

in men undergoing Transrectal prostate biopsy. Urology. 2012;**79**(1):32-36

[84] Hole J, Hirsch M, Ball E, Meads C. Music as an aid for postoperative recovery in adults: A systematic review and meta-analysis. The Lancet. 2015;**386**(10004):1659-1671

[85] Accardi MC, Milling LS. The effectiveness of hypnosis for reducing procedure-related pain in children and adolescents: A comprehensive methodological review. Journal of Behavioral Medicine. 2009;**32**(4): 328-339

Chapter 5

Perioperative Analgesia in Caesarean Section: What's New?

José Ramón Saucillo-Osuna, Eduardo Antonio Wilson-Manríquez, Mercedes Nicte López-Hernández and Ana Lilia Garduño-López

Abstract

Caesarean section is associated with moderate to severe postoperative pain during the first 24 hours after surgery. Inadequate pain management can influence recovery, maternal psychological well-being and breastfeeding. In the search of alternatives to minimize the use of systemic opioids, new recommendations have been made to implement protocols to improve recovery after caesarean section, with multimodal analgesia, new suggestions for neuraxial techniques, regional analgesia with ultrasound-guided fascial plane blocks and non-pharmacological approaches. Some of the interventions, such as epidural or spinal blocks, although effective, carry a significant risk of complications (for example post-puncture headache). In their place, newer alternatives such as interventions guided by ultrasound are safe and effective for relieving pain in this common clinical context. The goal of this chapter is to provide clinicians with up-to-date evidence for optimal pain management after elective caesarean section.

Keywords: caesarean section analgesia, pain after caesarean, multimodal analgesia, systemic opioids, regional blocks

1. Introduction

Caesarean section is the most performed surgical procedure in the world. This procedure is associated with moderate to severe postoperative pain during the first 24 hours after surgery. Inadequate pain management can influence recovery, maternal psychological well-being and breastfeeding. A core principle of successful postoperative analgesia is implementation of multimodal analgesia, and the caesarean section is no exception to the rule. The most effective and evidence-based intervention for effective postoperative analgesia for caesarean section is the use of neuraxial techniques such as epidural block, subarachnoid block or combined techniques, where morphine has played a fundamental role in analgesia in this surgery combined with non-steroidal anti-inflammatory drugs (NSAIDs) and acetaminophen [1]. However, there are multiple factors that may cause a patient to experience discomfort or pain during caesarean section, some of which are preventable and must certainly be

IntechOpen

Preoperative	Intraoperative	Postoperative	Surgical technique
• Intrathecal (IT) long-acting opioid morphine 50–100 μg or IT diamorphine (up to 300 μg) (Grade A). • Epidural morphine 1–3 mg or diamorphine up to 1–3 mg may be used as an alternative, for example, when an epidural catheter is used as part of a combined spinal-epidural technique (Grade A)	• Intravenous (IV) paracetamol if not administered pre-operatively (Grade A) • IV NSAIDs (Grade A) • IV dexamethasone (Grade A) • If IT morphine is not used, local anaesthetic wound infiltration (single-shot) or continuous wound infusion and/or regional analgesia techniques [fascial plane blocks such as transversus abdominis plane blocks and quadratus lumborum (QL) blocks] (Grade A)	• Oral or IV paracetamol (Grade A) • Oral or IV NSAIDs (Grade A) • Opioid for rescue or when other recommended strategies are not possible (e.g., contra-indications to regional anaesthesia) (Grade D) • Analgesic adjuncts include transcutaneous electrical nerve stimulation (TENS) (Grade A)	• Joel-Cohen incision (Grade A) • Non-closure of peritoneum (Grade A)

Adapted from Roofthooft et al. [2].

Table 1.
Overall recommendations for pain management in patients undergoing planned caesarean section.

managed. Therefore, knowing the updates on postoperative pain management in caesarean section gives us tools that allow us to manage pain in specific scenarios and individually. The most recent guidelines for the management of specific postoperative pain in caesarean section have been published by the Prospect Group [2], and their recommendations have been summarized in **Table 1**.

2. Multimodal analgesia

2.1 Acetaminophen

Acetaminophen is one of the most prescribed analgesics worldwide, it has an excellent safety profile and relatively few adverse effects. Its action mechanism for inhibiting acute postoperative pain has not been elucidated completely, however, it is believed to inhibit the cyclooxygenase (COX) enzyme and modulate the receptors Transient Receptor Potential Vanilloid 1 (TRPV1) and Cannabinoid 1 (CB1) in the midbrain, medulla and spinal cord which are mediators of pain modulation. It is usually administered via oral or IV routes, there is no difference in area under the curve and $t½$ between both routes, thereby being effective for analgesia in both presentations [3]. Recent guidelines establish that acetaminophen should be administered preoperatively (most easily oral), intraoperatively and should be continued in the postoperative period [4]. Established doses are 1000 mg every 6–8 hours, with a maximum established dose of 4000 mg per 24 hours [5].

2.2 Nonsteroidal anti-inflammatory drugs

NSAIDs are analgesic, antipyretic and anti-inflammatory drugs that inhibit the COX pathway of prostaglandin production [6]. Specifically, prostaglandin E2 and

F2a result in the sensitization of nociceptive nerve fibres to painful stimuli following tissue injury, NSAIDs cause a reduction in their synthesis and therefore analgesia [7]. There are no clear differences in analgesic efficacy between equipotent doses of different NSAIDs, the most used are ketorolac (IV) and ibuprofen (oral). These should be started in the intraoperative period (after delivery) and continued in the postoperative period. Their use in this patient population is well established, a meta-analysis by Zeng et al. [8] demonstrated that the perioperative use of NSAIDs in caesarean delivery patients resulted in significantly lower pain scores, less opioid consumption and less drowsiness/sedation.

2.3 Dexamethasone

Dexamethasone is a corticosteroid that has potent inhibitory effects on local inflammatory mediators and multiple pain pathways. It is a well-established antiemetic and is recommended in guidelines as prophylaxis for postoperative nausea and vomiting [9]. Recent evidence highlighted by a meta-analysis (that included multiple randomized control trials analysing patients having caesarean sections) reported a significant reduction in 24-hour morphine consumption and prolongation of time to first analgesic request with intraoperative dexamethasone use as part of a multi-modal analgesic regimen [10]. Dexamethasone does increase blood glucose but the clinical significance is small, caution should be exercised in patients with glucose intolerance or diabetes, and the risk for other adverse events after surgery is minimal [11]. The general recommendation is a single dose of 8–10 mg intraoperatively, higher doses have not been proven to be of added benefit [2].

2.4 Neuraxial analgesia

Neuraxial techniques are considered the cornerstone of pain management after caesarean section, since the relief reported by the patients compared to other techniques is superior. Kaufner et al. [12] compared three strategies of postoperative analgesia after caesarean section in 199 women who were randomized into three groups: the IT group, the epidural group and the patient-controlled epidural analgesia (PCEA) group. They reported analgesia less effective with PCEA (continuous infusion and epidural bolus controlled by the patient-PCEA of ropivacaine 0.1% bolus and sufentanil 0.5 mg/ml) compared with 3 mg epidural morphine and 0.1 mg spinal morphine in terms of pain relief. IT morphine had a better analgesic-sparing effect than epidural morphine. In this study, low dose and concentration of local anaesthetic in the PCEA group might explain this difference, and more evidence would be necessary to conclude.

However, recently in a systematic review [13] that included 54 randomized controlled trials (RCT) (3497 patients), the prevalence of inadequate neuraxial anaesthesia for elective caesarean section was 14.6% (95% CI 13.3–15.9%). The prevalence of conversion to general anaesthesia was 0.06% (95% CI 0.0–0.2%). Spinal/combined spinal-epidural anaesthesia was associated with a lower overall prevalence of inadequate neuraxial anaesthesia than epidural anaesthesia (10.2% vs. 30.3%, respectively) (95% CI 9.0–11.4% and 26.5–34.5%).

When the combined epidural-spinal block without morphine is selected as an anaesthetic strategy, it is always important to consider that the epidural may be insufficient for analgesia. Further management strategies are needed to optimize the treatment when inadequate or insufficient epidural analgesia occurs [1]. Pain after caesarean section under neuraxial anaesthesia represents a challenging clinical situation, where the anaesthesiologist will need to make swift decisions. It is important to explain to the woman possible rescue modalities if the neuraxial block is providing sub-optimal analgesia. Attention must be paid when the patient reports pain and an immediate change of plan must be made. A sensitivity test with pinprick and/or cold pressure should be performed during continuous anaesthetic local infusion. In case of insufficient analgesia (e.g. patched analgesia) the addition of epidural morphine or an opioid should be the first consideration. If the catheter does not work, the analgesic strategy may be the use of IV opioids or ultrasound-guided regional techniques [14].

Seki et al. [15] in 66 RCTs comprising 4400 patients undergoing caesarean section, compared with placebo, IT opioids (fentanyl, sufentanil and morphine) significantly prolonged the analgesia duration by 96, 96 and 190 minutes, respectively (mean difference). Although morphine ranked first, the efficacy of opioids was similar. Except for diamorphine, all opioids were associated with significant increases in the incidence of pruritus. Sufentanil and morphine were associated with increases in the incidence of respiratory depression. However, the use of IT or epidural morphine has been shown in several investigations to significantly optimize postoperative pain scores. Recently, the recommended dose of IT morphine has been reduced to 100 μg or lower doses resulting in adequate analgesia with fewer side effects [2, 16, 17]. Sharawi et al. [18] reported the safety of IT morphine for caesarean section with low incidence of respiratory depression, however, caution is especially required when IT morphine is used in morbidly obese patients. It is important to consider that morphine presents specific side effects (pruritus, nausea and/or vomiting) that may require specific monitoring, prophylaxis or interventions [19, 20]. The NICE guidelines have recommended IT diamorphine as an alternative to IT morphine. The dose spinal is 300 μg, and the epidural dose is 2–3 mg [2, 18, 21].

2.5 Regional blocks

2.5.1 Transverse abdominal plane block

The transverse abdominal plane (TAP) block involves injection of local anaesthetic into the fascia between the internal oblique muscle and transversus abdominis muscle, blocking the afferents of thoracolumbar nerves originating from the T6 to L1 spinal roots that run through the same fascia and innervate the anterolateral abdominal wall [22]. The safest and most efficient method of performing the TAP block is by real-time ultrasound guidance. A major disadvantage of the TAP block is that it doesn't provide visceral analgesia [23]. It is recommended as an analgesia adjunct of multimodal analgesia for patients having caesarean section and not receiving neuraxial morphine for any reason (e.g. general anaesthesia) [2]. The previous recommendation is based on information obtained from a recent meta-analysis, Champaneria et al. [24] state that TAP blocks significantly reduce pain and postoperative morphine consumption at rest both when compared with placebo or no TAP blocks, however, this significance is lost when compared to IT morphine or given in co-administration. Contrary to this, a recent network meta-analysis by Ryu et al. [25] concluded that combined IT morphine in conjunction with ilioinguinal–iliohypogastric nerve and anterior transversus abdominis plane block was the most effective post-caesarean analgesic strategy with lower rest pain at 6 hours and cumulative 24-hour morphine consumption. Additionally, other effective options for effective analgesia were IT morphine, ilioinguinal–iliohypogastric nerve block with IT morphine, lateral TAP block, and single shot or continuous wound infiltration (CWI). Ng et al. [26] analysed in a meta-analysis the difference between high-dose or low-dose local anaesthetic (bupivacaine equivalents >50 or ≤50 mg per block side, respectively) and demonstrated no difference in postoperative opioid consumption or pain scores after caesarean delivery. It is recommended to use low-dose local anaesthetic preparations for TAP blocks because of a lack of evidence of more effective analgesia with higher doses and to diminish the risk of local anaesthetic toxicity in this vulnerable patient population.

2.5.2 Quadratus lumborum block

The QL block involves the injection of local anaesthetic into one of three fascial planes adjacent to the QL muscle (anterior, middle or posterior layers) which comprise part of the thoracolumbar fascia (TLF). The action mechanism of this block is believed to be through blockade of nociceptive and sympathetic neurons that traverse the TLF and by a possible spread to the paravertebral space with somatic nerve and sympathetic trunk blockade [27, 28]. It is believed to provide somatic and visceral analgesia, usually between T7 and L1 dermatomes.

The QL block appears to be effective for postoperative analgesia after caesarean section. A recent meta-analysis de Tan et al. [29] found that in postoperative caesarean section, QL block reduced 24-hour opioid consumption (mean difference −10.64 mg morphine equivalents; -16.01 to -5.27), reduced dynamic pain at 6 hours and static pain and opioid consumption at 6 and 12 hours compared to controls.

Verma et al. compared the analgesic efficacy of QL block and TAP block after caesarean section. Their main findings were time for rescue analgesic requirement was significantly prolonged in patients with QL block (68.77 ± 1.74 hours) compared to patient with TAP block (13.3 ± 1.21 hours). The QL block group had significantly less analgesic demand ($P < 0.001$) at 2, 4, 6, 12, 24, 36, 48 and 72 hours postoperatively [30]. A more recent RCT compared the efficacy of ultrasound-guided TAP block and QL block on postoperative pain after caesarean section. The results favoured the efficacy of QL block with 15% of patients with QL block and 77% of patients with TAP block requiring rescue analgesia ($P < 0.001$). Significant differences in pain scores at 6, 8, 10, 12, 16 and 20 hours postoperatively, by 24 hours postoperatively the difference ceased to be statistically significant. Time to rescue analgesia in QL group was 1353 minutes (±224.07) and TAP group was 915 minutes (±391.62) ($P < 0.001$) [31]. Although evidence appeared promising that the QL block is more effective than the TAP block for postoperative pain after caesarean section, a recent meta-analysis found that QL block and TAP block were equivalent and superior in their analgesic efficacy relative to inactive control for up to 48 hours and that QL block was not associated with a reduction in 24-hour IV morphine equivalent consumption when compared with TAP block [32]. Recent guidelines recommend QL block as an option as part of a multi-modal analgesic strategy if IT morphine is not used [2].

2.5.3 Continuous wound infiltration

CWI is an analgesic technique that uses a multiorifice catheter placed at the surgical site and connected to an elastomeric infusion pump that delivers a constant, fixed-rate infusion of medications (usually local anaesthetics) to surrounding cutaneous nerves. For caesarean delivery, catheter placement is either between rectus fascia and subcutaneous tissue or deep into the fascia [23]. Many RCTs have demonstrated the benefit of this technique for postoperative analgesia. A recent randomized controlled double-blind study of 69 patients concluded that morphine consumption was significantly lower in the infusion group (21.52 mg ± 21.56) compared to the placebo group (29.57 mg ± 22.38; 95% CI [−18.8 to 2.76]; *P*-value = 0.047). No significant differences were observed in pain evaluated by visual analogue scale (VAS), except for pain at mobilization 6 hours after surgery (ropivacaine vs. placebo: 3.90 ± 2.66 vs. 5.36 ± 2.55; *P*-value = 0.030) [33]. Recent guidelines recommend CWI as an option as part of a multi-modal analgesic strategy if IT morphine is not used [2].

2.5.4 Erector spinae plane block

The erector spinae plane (ESP) block involves injection of local anaesthetic into the fascial plane of the TLF at the transverse process of the vertebrae [34]. The action mechanism is believed to be the spread of local anaesthetic through connective tissue and ligaments towards the costotransverse foramen and having a direct effect on the ventral and dorsal nerve roots of the spinal nerves corresponding to different thoracic segments. Another theory is blockade of communicating rami and the sympathetic chain to produce visceral analgesia [35].

Considering the probable visceral analgesia provided by the ESP block, it may have potential use in obstetric patients for postoperative analgesic management. In comparison with IT morphine for analgesia after elective caesarean delivery under spinal anaesthesia in an RCT [36], ESP block delayed the time to first analgesic request (4.93 ± 0.82 hours in the ITM group and 12 ± 2.81 hours in the ESP group) and significantly lowered tramadol consumption 101.7 ± 25.67 mg in IT morphine group, 44 ± 16.71 mg in ESP block group). This study also found significantly reduced VAS scores in the postoperative period (0–24 hours), however, the average reduction was 0.25 units which should not be considered clinically significant.

A recent meta-analysis [37] reported that there was no statistical difference in pain in the first 24 hours of the postoperative period when comparing ESP block to other interfascial blocks and IT morphine. However, ESP block showed a lower consumption of tramadol (mean difference = −47.66; 95% CI −77.24 to −18.08; I 2 = 59%; very low certainty) and longer blockade duration (mean difference = 6.97; 95% CI 6.30–7.65; I 2 = 58%; very low certainty), although the quality of evidence of these outcomes was very low.

A recent RCT [38] compared ESP block before induction of general anaesthesia for caesarean delivery versus conventional management with an IV analgesic regimen in the postoperative period. The ESP block group required less patient-controlled IV analgesia boluses ($P < 0.001$), had lower VAS scores and higher Bruggeman comfort scale scores at 2- and 6-hours postoperative intervals ($P < 0.05$), with no difference at 12 and 24 hours postoperative periods. The ESP block group also required less propofol and remifentanil ($P < 0.001$), had significantly shorter emergence time ($P = 0.003$) and less incidence of postoperative nausea and vomiting ($P = 0.014$). Recent guidelines recommend ESP block as an option as part of a multi-modal analgesic strategy if IT morphine is not used [2].

2.5.5 Ilioinguinal and iliohypogastric blocks

The ilioinguinal–iliohypogastric block has been shown to reduce postoperative opioid requirements after caesarean section; however, they apparently don't have benefits in postoperative analgesia compared with IT morphine [39–41]. Recently, Staker et al. [42] conducted a prospective, triple-blind, placebo-controlled randomized study of 100 women undergoing elective caesarean section. All women had spinal anaesthesia with hyperbaric bupivacaine, 15 μg fentanyl and 150 μg morphine, as well as 100 mg diclofenac and 1.5 g paracetamol rectally. Women were randomly allocated to receive the ilioinguinal–transversus abdominis plane block or a sham block at the end of surgery. The primary outcome was the difference in fentanyl patient-controlled analgesia (PCA) dose at 24 hours. Secondary outcomes included postoperative pain scores, adverse effects and maternal satisfaction. The cumulative mean (95%CI) fentanyl dose at 24 hours was 71.9 (55.6–92.7) μg in the ilioinguinal–transversus abdominis group compared with 179.1 (138.5–231.4) μg in the control group ($P < 0.001$). VAS scores averaged across time-points were 1.9 (1.5–2.3) millimetres (mm) vs. 5.0 (4.3–5.9) mm ($P = 0.006$) at rest and 4.7 (4.1–5.5) mm vs. 11.3 (9.9–13.0) mm ($P = 0.001$) on movement, respectively. Post-hoc analysis showed that the ilioinguinal–transversus abdominis group was less likely to use ≥1000 μg fentanyl compared with the control group (2% vs. 16%; $P = 0.016$). There were no differences in opioid-related side effects or maternal satisfaction with analgesia. The addition of the ilioinguinal–transversus abdominis plane block provides superior analgesia to usual multimodal analgesic regimen. More studies are needed to verify these data.

In the experience of the main author, after 48 hours of surgery, shortly before the discharge of the patient undergoing caesarean section (Pfannenstiel-type surgical wound), to complement oral analgesia at home, a bilateral ilioinguinal and iliohypogastric block is placed under ultrasound guidance, with 10 ml of 7.5% ropivacaine, this analgesic strategy achieves comfortable ambulation, low pain scores and analgesic savings.

2.6 Systemic opioids

When neuraxial analgesia or regional blocks for analgesia are not an option, oral or IV multi-modal analgesia strategy for postoperative pain management after caesarean delivery is implemented, a large percentage of patients will require systemic opioids. Oral or IV opioids should be used for rescue analgesia only, at the lowest effective dose and for the shortest duration possible. Oral opioids should be preferred over IV presentations if patients tolerate oral intake. A classic RCT [43] compared oral versus IV opioid strategy after caesarean delivery, demonstrating that oral opioid analgesia with oxycodone-paracetamol may offer superior pain control with less pain at 6 and 24 hours after the procedure ($P = 0.04$ and $P = 0.004$, respectively) and with fewer side-effects compared to morphine PCA. A practice advisory from the American College of Obstetricians and Gynecologists [44] advised that breastfeeding mothers should not receive codeine or tramadol based on evidence that the use of these medications in CYP2D6 ultra-metabolizers can result in excessive amounts of morphine in maternal breast milk with potential for neonatal overdose and respiratory depression. Instead, patients should receive oral oxycodone or hydromorphone. No individual drug has proven to be superior in terms of analgesia or side-effect profile when compared with any other opioid [2]. Due to considerations of continuous breastfeeding, in case of requirement of IV opioids for postoperative analgesia, morphine is the recommended choice based on reliable clinical effects and proven safety [21, 44]. Offer oral morphine sulphate to women. If the patient cannot take oral medication (for example, because of nausea or vomiting), offer IV morphine. Consider IV PCA using morphine for women who have had a general anaesthetic for caesarean birth. If IV PCA is not acceptable to the woman, or the pain is less severe, consider oral morphine sulphate [21].

2.7 Non-pharmacological interventions

TENS is a non-invasive peripheral stimulation technique used to relieve pain. Some publications have shown a beneficial effect of TENS as a treatment or as a rescue strategy, in addition to the fact that patients report more satisfaction with its use [45, 46].

Surgical strategies that have been shown to reduce pain scores are the Joel-Cohen incision and non-closure of the peritoneum [47–49].

On the other hand, music therapy has been shown to reduce the physiological and cognitive responses of anxiety in patients undergoing caesarean section [50].

3. Conclusions

Providing adequate analgesia after a caesarean section confers advantages in the mother-child relationship. The combination of NSAIDs, paracetamol and neuraxial techniques with IT morphine or diamorphine is considered the cornerstone of analgesic management. However, new regional ultrasound-guided techniques have now emerged, such as TAP block, QL block, ESP block, ilioinguinal and iliohypogastric among others, which in a multimodal context also favour adequate pain relief. The use of opioids is reserved as analgesic rescue in combination with the previously mentioned techniques or for those patients who are not candidates for neuraxial or regional techniques, where the minimum effective doses of opioids are recommended. Finally, the use of non-pharmacological strategies is not yet widespread in hospitals, although some techniques such as music and tens seem to be effective.

Conflict of interest

The authors declare no conflict of interest.

Author details

José Ramón Saucillo-Osuna[1], Eduardo Antonio Wilson-Manríquez[2], Mercedes Nicte López-Hernández[3] and Ana Lilia Garduño-López[2]*

1 Bluenet Hospitals, Cabo San Lucas, BCS, México

2 Instituto Nacional de Ciencias Médicas y Nutrición Salvador Zubirán, CDMX, México

3 Hospital Angeles Interlomas, CDMX, México

*Address all correspondence to: ana.gardunol@incmnsz.mx

References

[1] Landau R, Janvier A. Are we finally tackling the issue of pain during cesarean section? Anaesthesia Critical Care and Pain Medicine. 2021;**40**:100938

[2] Roofthooft E, Joshi G, Rawal N, Van de Velde M, PROSPECT Working Group of the European Society of Regional Anaesthesia and Pain Therapy and supported by the Obstetric Anaesthetists' Association. PROSPECT guideline for elective caesarean section: updated systematic review and procedure-specific postoperative pain management recommendations. Anaesthesia. 2021;**76**(5):665-680

[3] Ohashi N, Kohno T. Analgesic effect of acetaminophen: A review of known and novel mechanisms of action. Frontiers in Pharmacology. 30 Nov 2020;**11**:580289

[4] Patel K, Zakowski M. Enhanced recovery after cesarean: current and emerging trends. Current Anesthesiology Reports. 2021;**11**(2):136-144

[5] FDA. Acetaminophen information. Food Drug Admin. 2017. Available from: https://www.fda.gov/drugs/information-drug-class/acetaminophen-information

[6] Sangkum L, Thamjamrassri T, Arnuntasupakul V, Chalacheewa T. The current consideration, approach, and management in postcesarean delivery pain control: a narrative review. Anesthesiology Research and Practice. 2021;**2021**:2156918

[7] Bosch DJ, Nieuwenhuijs-Moeke GJ, van Meurs M, Abdulahad WH, Struys MMRF. Immune modulatory effects of nonsteroidal anti-inflammatory drugs in the perioperative period and their consequence on postoperative outcome. Anesthesiology. 2022;**136**(5):843-860

[8] Zeng AM, Nami NF, Wu CL, Murphy JD. The analgesic efficacy of nonsteroidal anti-inflammatory agents (NSAIDs) in patients undergoing cesarean deliveries: a meta-analysis. Regional Anesthesia and Pain Medicine. 2016;**41**(6):763-772

[9] Gan TJ, Belani KG, Bergese S, Chung F, Diemunsch P, Habib AS, et al. Fourth consensus guidelines for the management of postoperative nausea and vomiting. Anesthesia and Analgesia. 2020;**131**(2):411-448

[10] Heesen M, Rijs K, Hilber N, Eid K, Al-Oweidi A, Rossaint R, et al. Effect of intravenous dexamethasone on postoperative pain after spinal anaesthesia - a systematic review with meta-analysis and trial sequential analysis. Anaesthesia. 2019;**74**(8):1047-1056

[11] Myles P, Corcoran T. Benefits and risks of dexamethasone in noncardiac surgery. Anesthesiology. 2021;**135**:895-903. DOI: 10.1097/ALN.0000000000003898

[12] Kaufner L, Heimann S, Zander D, Weizsäcker K, Correns I, Sander M, et al. Neuraxial anesthesia for pain contro after cesarean section: a prospective randomized trial comparing three different neuraxial techniques in clinical practice. Minerva Anestesiologica. 2016;**82**:514-524

[13] Kim WH, Hur M, Park SK, Yoo S, Lim T, Yoon HK, et al. Comparison between general, spinal, epidural, and combined spinal-epidural anesthesia

for cesarean delivery: A network meta-analysis. International Journal of Obstetric Anesthesia. 2019;**37**:5-15

[14] Veef E, Van de Velde M. Post-cesarean section analgesia. Best Practice & Research. Clinical Anaesthesiology. 2022;**36**(1):83-88

[15] Seki H, Shiga T, Mihara T, Hoshijima H, Hosokawa Y, Hyuga S, et al. Effects of intrathecal opioids on cesarean section: a systematic review and Bayesian network meta-analysis of randomized controlled trials. Journal of Anesthesia. 2021;**35**:911-927

[16] Sultan P, Halpern SH, Pushpanathan E, Patel S, Carvalho B. The effect of intrathecal morphine dose on outcomes after elective Cesarean delivery: a meta-analysis. Anesthesia and Analgesia. 2016;**123**:154-164

[17] Berger JS, Gonzalez A, Hopkins A, Alshaeri T, Jeon D, Wang S, et al. Dose-response of intrathecal morphine when administered with intravenous ketorolac for post-cesarean analgesia: a two-center, prospective, randomized, blinded trial. International Journal of Obstetric Anesthesia. 2016;**28**:3-11

[18] Sharawi N, Carvalho B, Habib AS, Blake L, Jm M, Sultan P. A systematic review evaluating neuraxial morphine and diamorphine associated respiratory depression after Cesarean delivery. Anesthesia and Analgesia. 2018;**127**:1385-1395

[19] Dominguez JE, Habib AS. Prophylaxis and treatment of the side-effects of neuraxial morphine analgesia following cesarean delivery. Current Opinion in Anaesthesiology. 2013;**26**(3):288-295

[20] Waxler B, Dadabhoy ZP, Stojiljkovic l, Rabito S. Primer of postoperative pruritus for anesthesiologists. Anesthesiology. 2005;**103**:168-178

[21] National Institute for Health and Care Excellence. 2021 Opioid for pain relief after caesarean birth. NICE Guideline No. 192. Available from: https://www.nice.org.uk/guidance/ng192/evidence/f-opioids-for-pain-relief-after-caesarean-birth-pdf-9071941651

[22] Tsai HC, Yoshida T, Chuang TY, Yang SF, Chang CC, Yao HY, et al. Transversus abdominis plane block: an updated review of anatomy and techniques. BioMed Research International. 2017;**2017**:8284363

[23] Mitchell KD, Smith CT, Mechling C, Wessel CB, Orebaugh S, Lim G. A review of peripheral nerve blocks for cesarean delivery analgesia. Regional Anesthesia and Pain Medicine. 25 Oct 2019:rapm-2019-100752

[24] Champaneria R, Shah L, Wilson MJ, Daniels JP. Clinical effectiveness of transversus abdominis plane (TAP) blocks for pain relief after caesarean section: a meta-analysis. International Journal of Obstetric Anesthesia. 2016;**28**:45-60

[25] Ryu C, Choi GJ, Jung YH, Baek CW, Cho CK, Kang H. Postoperative analgesic effectiveness of peripheral nerve blocks in cesarean delivery: a systematic review and network meta-analysis. Journal of Personalized Medicine. 2022;**12**(4):634

[26] Ng SC, Habib AS, Sodha S, Carvalho B, Sultan P. High-dose versus low-dose local anaesthetic for transversus abdominis plane block post-Caesarean delivery analgesia: a meta-analysis. British Journal of Anaesthesia. 2018;**120**(2):252-263

[27] Elsharkawy H, El-Boghdadly K, Barrington M. Quadratus Lumborum block: anatomical concepts, mechanisms, and techniques. Anesthesiology. 2019;**130**(2):322-335

[28] Akerman M, Pejčić N, Veličković I. A review of the quadratus lumborum block and ERAS. Frontiers in Medicine. 2018;**5**:44. DOI: 10.3389/fmed.2018.00044

[29] Tan HS, Taylor C, Weikel D, Barton K, Habib AS. Quadratus lumborum block for postoperative analgesia after cesarean delivery: a systematic review with meta-analysis and trial-sequential analysis. Journal of Clinical Anesthesia. 2020;**67**:110003

[30] Verma K, Malawat A, Jethava D, Jethava DD. Comparison of transversus abdominis plane block and quadratus lumborum block for post-caesarean section analgesia: a randomised clinical trial. Indian Journal of Anaesthesia. 2019;**63**(10):820-826

[31] Khanna S, Krishna Prasad GV, Sharma VJ, Biradar M, Bhasin D. Quadratus lumborum block versus transversus abdominis plane block for post Caesarean analgesia: a randomized prospective controlled study. Medical Journal, Armed Forces India. 2022;**78**(Suppl. 1):S82-S88. DOI: 10.1016/j.mjafi.2020.10.009

[32] El-Boghdadly K, Desai N, Halpern S, Blake L, Odor PM, Bampoe S, et al. Quadratus lumborum block vs. transversus abdominis plane block for caesarean delivery: a systematic review and network meta-analysis. Anaesthesia. 2021;**76**(3):393-403

[33] Rosetti J, Francotte J, Noel E, Drakopoulos P, Rabbachin N, de Brucker M. Continuous ropivacaine subfascial wound infusion after cesarean delivery in pain management: a prospective randomized controlled double-blind study. International Journal of Gynaecology and Obstetrics. 2021;**154**(1):79-84

[34] Forero M, Adhikary SD, Lopez H, Tsui C, Chin KJ. The erector spinae plane block: a novel analgesic technique in thoracic neuropathic pain. Regional Anesthesia and Pain Medicine. 2016;**41**(5):621-627

[35] Yang HM, Choi YJ, Kwon HJ, O J, Cho TH, Kim SH. Comparison of injectate spread and nerve involvement between retrolaminar and erector spinae plane blocks in the thoracic region: a cadaveric study. Anaesthesia. 2018;**73**(10):1244-124

[36] Hamed MA, Yassin HM, Botros JM, Abdelhady MA. Analgesic efficacy of erector spinae plane block compared with intrathecal morphine after elective cesarean section: a prospective randomized controlled study. Journal of Pain Research. 2020;**13**:597-604

[37] Ribeiro Junior IDV, Carvalho VH, Brito LGO. Erector spinae plane block for analgesia after cesarean delivery: a systematic review with meta-analysis. Brazilian Journal of Anesthesiology. 2022;**72**(4):506-515

[38] Hu J, Chen Q, Xu Q, Song Y, Wei K, Lei XF. Analgesic effect of ultrasound-guided erector spinae plane block (espb) in general anesthesia for cesarean section: a randomized controlled trial. BMC Anesthesiology. 2022;**22**(1):244

[39] Al-Dehayat G, Al-Momany M. Ilioinguinal-Iliohyogastric peripheral nerve block for analgesia after caesarean section. Journal of the Royal Medical Services. 2008;**15**:70-72

[40] Sakalli M, Ceyhan A, Uysal HY, Yazici I, Başar H. The efficacy of ilioinguinal and iliohypogastric nerve block for postoperative pain after caesarean section. Journal of Research in Medical Sciences. 2010;**15**:6-13

[41] Vallejo MC, Steen TL, Cobb BT, et al. Efficacy of the bilateral

ilioinguinal-iliohypogastric block with intrathecal morphine for postoperative cesarean delivery analgesia. Scientific World Journal. 2012;**2012**:107316

[42] Staker JJ, Liu D, Church R, Carlson DJ, Panahkhahi M, Lim A, et al. A triple-blind, placebo-controlled randomised trial of the ilioinguinal-transversus abdominis plane (I-TAP) nerve block for elective caesarean section. Anaesthesia. 2018;**73**(5):594-602

[43] Davis KM, Esposito MA, Meyer BA. Oral analgesia compared with intravenous patient-controlled analgesia for pain after cesarean delivery: a randomized controlled trial. American Journal of Obstetrics and Gynecology. 2006;**194**(4):967-971

[44] http://www.acog.org/About-ACOG/News-Room/Practice-Advisories/PracticeAdvisory-on-Codeine-and-Tramadol-for-Breastfeeding-Women. April 27th 2017

[45] Khooshideh M, Latifi Rostami SS, Sheikh M, Ghorbani Yekta B, Shahriari A. Pulsed electromagnetic fields for postsurgical pain management in women undergoing cesarean section: a randomized, double-blind, placebo-controlled trial. The Clinical Journal of Pain. 2017;**33**(2):142-114

[46] Chakravarthy M, Prashanth A, George A. Evaluation of percutaneous electrical nerve stimulation of the auricleor relief of postoperative pain following cesarean section. Medical Acupuncture. 2019;**31**:281e8

[47] Kurek Eken M, Özkaya E, Tarhan T, İçöz Ş, Eroğlu Ş, Kahraman ŞT, et al. Effects of closure versus non-closure of the visceral and parietal peritoneum at cesarean section: does it have any effect on postoperative vital signs? A prospective randomized study. Journal of Maternal-Fetal & Neonatal Medicine. 2017;**30**(8):922-926

[48] Omran EF, Meshaal H, Hassan SM, Dieb AS, Nabil H, Saad H. The effect of rectus muscle re-approximation at cesarean delivery on pain perceived after operation: a randomized control trial. Journal of Maternal-Fetal & Neonatal Medicine. 2019;**32**(19):3238-3243

[49] Bamigboye AA, Hofmeyr GJ. Closure versus non-closure of the peritoneum at caesarean section: short- and long-term outcomes. Cochrane Database of Systematic Reviews. 2014;**8**:CD000163

[50] Handan E, Sahiner NC, Bal MD, Dissiz M. Effects of music during multiple cesarean section delivery. Journal of the College of Physicians and Surgeons–Pakistan. 2018;**28**(3):247-249

Chapter 6

Postoperative Pain in Pediatrics

Alejandro Escalona-Espinosa, Kelly Maldonado-Sánchez, Enrique Pazos-Alvarado, Pedro Castañeda, Rosina Alcaraz-Ramos, David Aguilar-Romero and Keisuke Lira-Hernandez

Abstract

Postoperative pain in pediatrics is a common concern for both parents and healthcare professionals. Children who experience pain after surgery can present with several complications, including nausea, vomiting, breathing difficulties, sleep disturbances, and decreased physical activity. In addition, untreated pain can have long-term effects on children's emotional and psychological well-being. It is important to recognize that children may experience pain differently than adults and, therefore, need a personalized treatment approach. Evaluation and management of postoperative pain in pediatrics should be based on the child's age, the type of surgery, and the severity of pain. Several treatment options are available, including oral, intravenous, and epidural analgesics, as well as non-pharmacological techniques such as relaxation and distraction. Prevention of postoperative pain is also important and can be achieved through the administration of analgesics prior to surgery and early postoperative care.

Keywords: postoperative pain, pediatrics, analgesia, pain management, pain treatment

1. Introduction

Surgery is a common medical procedure performed to treat various conditions. In pediatrics, surgery is often necessary to treat congenital diseases, developmental disorders, or traumatic injuries. Although surgery can be beneficial, postoperative pain is a common consequence that can negatively affect a patient's recovery. Treatment may include pain relievers, regional anesthesia, and nondrug therapies such as physical therapy and occupational therapy. Within the strategies to prevent postoperative pain, such as the use of less invasive surgical techniques and the administration of analgesics before surgery. A multidisciplinary approach to postoperative pain management in pediatric patients, involving physicians, nurses, physiotherapists, and occupational therapists helps improve the conditions of pediatric patients after surgery. The importance of education and preparation to the patients and their parents before surgery helps to reduce anxiety and stress. It is also useful to implement relaxation and distraction techniques to improve the patient experience as well as the importance of using multimodal analgesia in pain management. In summary, in this chapter, we will highlight the importance of proper postoperative pain management in pediatric patients to minimize discomfort and promote a faster and more complete recovery.

In summary, in this chapter, we will highlight the importance of proper postoperative pain management in pediatric patients to minimize discomfort and promote a faster and more complete recovery.

2. Causes of postoperative pain in pediatrics

The causes of postoperative pain in children are multiple and may vary depending on the type of surgery. Some common causes may include tissue inflammation, manipulation of organs during surgery, surgical incision, and muscle strain associated with the recovery process. In addition, postoperative pain can also be caused by psychological factors. Some of the common causes of postoperative pain in pediatrics include:

- Tissue damage: Surgery can cause tissue damage, which can trigger an inflammatory response in the body and lead to pain.
- Invasive procedures: Invasive procedures, such as the insertion of drainage tubes or the placement of intravenous lines, can cause pain.
- Surgical incision: The surgical incision can be painful and take time to heal.
- Anxiety: Anxiety and fear can increase the perception of pain in children.

3. Symptoms of postoperative pain in pediatrics

Postoperative pain in pediatrics can manifest itself in different ways, and the symptoms may vary depending on the age of the patient and the nature of the surgery. Some of the common symptoms of postoperative pain in pediatrics include:

- Inconsolable crying.
- Irritability or restlessness.
- Refusal to eat or drink.
- Difficulty to sleep.
- Changes in heart and respiratory rate.
- Excessive sweating.
- Changes in facial expressions such as frowning or closing your eyes.
- Fetal position or muscle tension.
- Changes in physical activity or movement patterns.
- Changes in urination and bowel movements.

Pain identification in pediatrics can be challenging, especially in young children or those who cannot communicate verbally. In older children, there may be verbal reports of pain, as well as facial and bodily responses to painful stimuli. It is important that healthcare professionals working with children are trained in pain assessment and use appropriate assessment tools based on the child's age and development to ensure accurate identification of pain [1].

4. Treatment of postoperative pain in pediatrics

It is important to treat postoperative pain in pediatrics effectively to minimize discomfort and promote faster recovery, so some of the challenges associated with managing postoperative pain in children, including the lack of objective measures to assess pain, the variability in individual response to pain, and the need to balance the efficacy of treatment with potential side effects. It is important to explore various strategies to overcome these challenges such as the use of validated pain scales, personalization of treatment, and continuing education of healthcare personnel [2]. Treatment of postoperative pain in pediatrics may include a combination of pharmacological and non-pharmacological techniques. Some common treatment options include:

- Validated pain scales: The use of validated pain scales is suggested to assess postoperative pain in children such as the face scale, the numerical scale, or the color scale. These tools can help assess pain level and guide appropriate intervention.

- Multimodal analgesia: The use of a combination of analgesics and techniques is recommended to address different aspects of postoperative pain in children. This may include the use of opioid and non-opioid analgesics, peripheral nerve blocks, local infiltration, or epidural infusions.

- Relaxation and distraction techniques: Relaxation and distraction techniques, such as music, games, and virtual reality therapy, are suggested to help patients manage pain and anxiety.

- Education and preoperative preparation: The importance of educating patients and their families on postoperative pain management and providing preoperative preparation to reduce anxiety and improve postoperative recovery is highlighted.

- Treatment personalization: It is recommended to personalize treatment for each patient based on their individual needs and response to pain.

In addition to these treatment options, it is important that parents and medical staff work together to create a calm and comfortable environment for the patient.

Multimodal analgesia may include a combination of different drug classes such as nonsteroidal anti-inflammatory drugs (NSAIDs), opioids, local anesthetics, and gabapentinoids [3]. Drug selection and dosage must be individualized according to the needs of the patient. Furthermore, the choice of regional anesthesia technique may also influence the selection of multimodal analgesia. Regional anesthesia, such as epidural anesthesia or intravenous regional anesthesia, selectively blocks pain transmission from peripheral nerves to the spinal cord and brain, which may reduce the need for opioids and minimize opioid-associated side effects. In addition, regional anesthesia can reduce inflammation and the body's inflammatory response, which can help prevent chronic postoperative pain [4].

Some of the most commonly used NSAIDs in pediatrics include:

- Ibuprofen: It is one of the most commonly used NSAIDs in pediatrics due to its efficacy and safety. It is used to treat pain, inflammation, and fever. It is available in different formulations, including tablets, oral suspension, and rectal suppositories. The recommended dose is 5–10 mg/kg/dose, with an interval of 6–8 hours between each dose.

- Diclofenac: It is another NSAID that is used in pediatrics to treat pain and inflammation. It is available in different formulations, including tablets, rectal suppositories, and topical gel. In general, the recommended dose of diclofenac in children is 1–3 mg/kg/day, divided into 2–3 daily doses.

- Naproxen: It is an NSAID used to treat pain, inflammation, and fever in pediatrics. It is available in different formulations, including tablets and oral suspension. The recommended dose of naproxen in children is 5–10 mg/kg/dose every 12 hours, or 10–15 mg/kg/dose every 24 hours for the extended-release formulation.

- Paracetamol: This analgesic is not an NSAID. It is usually given as an oral suspension, and the recommended dose varies according to the age and weight of the child. In general, the recommended dose for children is 10–15 mg/kg/dose, with an interval of 4–6 hours between each dose. It is important not to exceed the maximum recommended dose.

It is important to note that NSAIDs can have side effects such as gastric irritation, gastric ulcers, and kidney problems, so they should be used with caution and under the supervision of a physician. Also, each patient may react differently to medications, so it is important to adjust the dose and treatment regimen individually for each child [5].

The use of opioids in pediatrics is used to control moderate to severe pain in children and adolescents. However, their use must be carefully supervised by a doctor as they can have serious and potentially dangerous side effects. Opioids are used in situations where non-opioid pain relievers are not enough to control pain. They can be used for the management of postoperative pain, cancer pain, and pain associated with chronic diseases [6]. It is important to note that prolonged use of opioids in children and adolescents may increase the risk of developing dependence and addiction. Therefore, steps should be taken to reduce the amount of opioids used and their duration, in order to minimize the risk of long-term health problems.

There are different opioids that can be used in pediatrics, some of them are:

- Hydrocodone: It is recommended to start with the lowest possible dose and adjust the dose as necessary to achieve effective pain control without causing serious side effects. The recommended dose is 0.05–0.2 mg/kg every 4–6 hours as needed, with an upper limit of 5 mg per dose and 20 mg in 24 hours in children 6–12 years of age. In children over 12 years of age, the recommended dose is 2.5–10 mg every 4–6 hours as needed, with a maximum limit of 40 mg in 24 hours.

- Fentanyl: It can be administered by different routes, including intravenous, epidural, intrathecal, or transdermal, depending on the clinical situation of the patient. The recommended dose is 1–2 mcg/kg, administered intravenously, every 2–4 hours as needed.

- Morphine: It can be administered orally, intravenously, subcutaneously, epidurally, or intrathecally, depending on the clinical situation of the patient. The recommended starting dose is 0.1–0.2 mg/kg every 4 hours intravenously or every 6 hours orally. However, the dosage may vary depending on the condition of the patient and the severity of the pain.

- Buprenorphine: Unlike other opioids, buprenorphine has a ceiling effect, which means that its pain-relieving effect levels off at higher doses and does not increase beyond a certain point, reducing the risk of overdose. Additionally, buprenorphine has lower addiction potential and respiratory side effects compared to other opioids. The recommended dose in pediatrics ranges between 10 and 20 mcg/kg/dose every 6–8 hours. However, these doses may vary based on the weight and age of the child and may be adjusted as needed to achieve adequate pain control.

- Tramadol: It is important to note that the use of tramadol in pediatrics requires careful assessment of the benefit–risk balance, especially in children under 12 years of age and in those with risk factors for opioid-related adverse events. The recommended dose of tramadol is 1–2 mg/kg/dose, administered, orally every 4–6 hours as needed. The maximum daily dose should not exceed 8 mg/kg/day.

It is important to emphasize that the use of opioids in pediatrics must be carefully supervised by a physician since they can have serious and potentially dangerous side effects such as respiratory depression or excessive sedation. In addition, the dose and duration of treatment should be appropriate to the child's age and weight, and measures should be taken to reduce the amount of opioids used and their duration, in order to minimize the risk of dependence and long-term health problems.

Gabapentinoids, such as gabapentin and pregabalin, are also used in pediatrics for pain management. However, the evidence on its safety and efficacy in children is limited, and more studies are needed to determine its appropriate use in this population. Some studies have found that pregabalin may be effective for neuropathic pain in children and adolescents, but more research is needed in this field. Also, caution should be exercised when using gabapentinoids in children with kidney problems as these drugs are primarily eliminated by the kidneys [7].

The best option to decide pain management in pediatrics is the analgesic ladder. The pediatric analgesic ladder is based on the World Health Organization (WHO) initiative for pain management in adult cancer patients. In 1986, the WHO proposed a guideline for pain management in adults with cancer, which became the WHO Analgesic Ladder in 1986. Later, in 1990, the WHO extended the analgesic ladder to include pain management in pediatric patients with cancer. Since then, the WHO analgesic ladder has become a standard guideline for pain management in pediatric and adult patients worldwide [8].

This staircase is divided into three levels:

- Level I: Non-opioid pain relievers (e.g., acetaminophen and ibuprofen).
- Level II: Mild to moderate opioid pain relievers (e.g., tramadol).
- Level III: Strong opioid pain relievers (e.g., morphine, fentanyl).

The idea is to start at the bottom of the ladder and work your way up as necessary to control the patient's pain. It is important to note that analgesic selection should be based on the etiology of the pain and the age and weight of the patient, and that the dose and frequency should be individually adjusted [9].

Within the non-pharmacological alternatives for pain management, we can find psychological intervention. For this type of treatment, the importance of accurate assessment and diagnosis of the cause of the pain is paramount since there are different psychological approaches such as cognitive behavioral therapy, acceptance and commitment therapy, interpersonal therapy, and family therapy. There is evidence that suggests that these therapies can be effective in the management of chronic and recurrent pain in children and adolescents, improving the quality of life, functionality, and psychological well-being of patients. However, there are also limitations of psychological therapies such as:

- Lack of high-quality studies: Although there are studies on psychological therapies in the management of chronic and recurrent pain in children and adolescents, many of them have methodological and design limitations, which limit the quality of the evidence.
- Heterogeneity in interventions: Psychological interventions include a variety of approaches and techniques, making it difficult to compare their effectiveness and determine, which is most appropriate for each patient.
- Lack of studies on specific populations: Most studies have been conducted in children and adolescents with chronic abdominal pain or headache, limiting the generalizability of the results to other populations.
- Difficulties in implementation: The implementation of psychological therapies can be expensive and require the training of specialized professionals, which limits their accessibility and availability in some health care settings.

However, more research is needed to determine the effectiveness of specific therapies for different types of pain: chronic and recurrent in specific populations of children and adolescents. To establish the best strategies for the implementation and integration of psychological treatments in pediatric medical care [10].

5. Prevention of postoperative pain in pediatrics

Although pediatric postoperative pain is often unavoidable, there are measures that can be taken to minimize its intensity and duration. Some strategies to prevent postoperative pain in pediatrics include:

- Use of less invasive surgical techniques.
- Use of regional anesthesia instead of general anesthesia.
- Administration of analgesics before surgery to prevent pain.
- Education and preparation of the patient and their parents before surgery to reduce anxiety and stress.

One of the methods most used by anesthesiologists is anesthetic adjuvants, which are drugs that are used in combination with local or general anesthetics to improve the efficacy of anesthesia and reduce postoperative pain [11]. In pediatrics, various anesthetic adjuvants are used to prevent postoperative pain, including:

- Clonidine: It is an alpha-2 adrenergic agonist that is used as an analgesic and sedative. Clonidine has been shown to reduce the need for opioid pain relievers after surgery in children. From 1 to 17 years, 2–5 micrograms/kg administered 30–60 minutes before the procedure, not to exceed the dose of 300 micrograms.
- Ketamine: It is a dissociative anesthetic that has analgesic and anesthetic properties. Ketamine has been shown to reduce postoperative pain and decrease the need for opioids in children. The dose for induction of anesthesia in healthy children is usually 1–2 mg/kg administered intravenously (IV), although it may vary according to the age and health status of the child, as well as the duration and type of procedure. For continuous infusion during surgery, the doses may be lower (0.25–0.5 mg/kg/hour).
- Dexmedetomidine: It is a clonidine-like alpha-2 adrenergic agonist used as an analgesic and sedative. Dexmedetomidine has been shown to be effective in reducing postoperative pain in children. In general, it is started with a low dose and gradually increased as needed. It is recommended that the dose of dexmedetomidine not exceed 1.5 mcg/kg/h in children. The following is a general formula for calculating the dose of pediatric dexmedetomidine:

Dexmedetomidine dose (mcg/kg/h) = body weight (kg) × starting dose (mcg/kg/h) × adjustment factor.

The adjustment factor varies according to the age of the child:
< 6 months: adjustment factor of 0.4.
6 months - 5 years: adjustment factor of 0.5.

- Magnesium: Magnesium has been shown to have pain-relieving properties and reduces the need for opioid pain relievers in children after surgery. In general, for the administration of IV magnesium in pediatrics, the recommended dose is

25 to 50 mg/kg, diluted in 5% saline or dextrose solution, at an infusion rate not greater than 150 mg/minute.

- Lidocaine: In addition to its use as a local anesthetic, lidocaine has been used as an anesthetic adjuvant to reduce postoperative pain in children. In regional epidural anesthesia, the dose of lidocaine is generally calculated based on the weight of the child, with a typical dose of 1–2 mg/kg. In local anesthesia, the maximum recommended dose is 4.5 mg/kg, and it can be reduced depending on the weight and age of the child.

Anesthetic adjuvants may offer several benefits in children, including:

1. Postoperative pain reduction: Anesthetic adjuvants, such as lidocaine or dexmedetomidine, may help reduce postoperative pain in children. This can improve children's quality of life after surgery and reduce the need for strong pain relievers.

2. Anxiety and stress reduction: Some anesthetic adjuvants, such as clonidine or midazolam, can help reduce anxiety and stress in children before surgery. This can make the process less scary and more manageable for the child.

3. Fewer side effects: Anesthetic adjuvants can help reduce the amount of general anesthetic needed for surgery, which can reduce side effects, such as nausea and vomiting.

4. Shorter recovery time: Some anesthetic adjuvants, such as dexmedetomidine, can help speed recovery time after surgery in children. This can reduce the need for a long hospital stay and help the child return to normal activities more quickly.

It is important to keep in mind that each child is different, and that the benefits of anesthetic adjuvants may vary depending on the case.

Another of the most widely used and recommended methods for postoperative pain management are non-pharmacological techniques, for example, stress and anxiety reduction. Strategies to reduce anxiety and stress in children before surgery can help prevent postoperative pain in several ways. First, by reducing anxiety and stress, the sensation of pain and the perception of its intensity can be reduced. Additionally, these techniques can help reduce the need for pain relievers and other postoperative pain medications, which can decrease the risk of side effects and complications. In addition, some techniques, such as muscle relaxation and meditation, can help improve sleep quality and reduce postoperative insomnia [12].

Some strategies that can help reduce anxiety and stress in these children include:

- Clear and precise information about the procedure: It is important that the child understands what will happen before, during, and after the surgical procedure. This can help to reduce anxiety and stress.

- Play therapy: Playful games and activities can be an effective way to reduce anxiety and stress in children facing a surgical procedure.

- Relaxation techniques: Relaxation techniques, such as deep breathing and visualization, can help reduce anxiety and stress in children.

- Use of antianxiety medications: Some antianxiety medications can help reduce anxiety and stress in children before the surgical procedure.

It is important that any strategy to reduce anxiety and stress in children who will undergo surgery is discussed with the medical team and that the most appropriate option is chosen for each child.

6. Scales to assess pain in children

Pain assessment in children can be challenging as children may have difficulty communicating their pain effectively. Therefore, it is important to use specific tools for pain assessment in children [13]. Some of these tools include:

- Numerical scales: These scales consist of the child assigning a number from 1 to 10 to indicate the intensity of his pain. Number scales are useful for older children who can count and understand number relationships.

- Face scales: These scales show a series of pictures that represent different levels of pain. The child chooses the drawing that best represents the intensity of her pain.

- Coloring scales: These scales consist of a drawing that the child must color according to the location and intensity of the pain.

- Behavioral rating scales: These scales assess the child's behavior rather than his verbal self-report. They are used for very young children who cannot yet communicate verbally.

- Structured clinical interviews: These interviews use specific questions to assess pain in children. They are used for children who have difficulty communicating their pain effectively.

- Among the most useful scales to assess pain in children who cannot communicate verbally such as infants or children with cognitive disabilities, as well as to standardize pain assessment in clinical and research situations, we can find the following:

- Wong-Baker faces scale: uses drawings of faces for the child to choose the one that best represents their pain, from a smiling face without pain to a crying face in pain.

- Numerical scale: The child is asked to assign a number from 0 to 10 to indicate the intensity of their pain, with zero being no pain and 10 being the most intense pain imaginable.

- Visual analog scale (VAS): A line is used that goes from one end indicating "no pain" to the other end indicating "unbearable pain," and the child is asked to mark on the line the point that best represents their pain.

- McGill face scale: uses a series of pictures that represent different types of pain such as stabbing, cutting, burning, etc. The child selects the pictures that describe his/her pain.

It is important to note that no tool is perfect for all children and situations. Selecting the right tool for the child and his/her specific situation will help us to better identify the situation. In addition, it must be taken into account that the evaluation of pain in children must be continuous and adapted as the child grows and develops new communication skills.

In addition, the use of scales to assess pain in children allows health professionals to obtain information on the intensity, duration, and location of pain, which can be useful for adjusting treatment and for long-term follow-up. It also allows parents and caregivers to more accurately communicate the symptoms the child is experiencing, which can help improve the child's care and quality of life.

It must be considered that the scales to assess pain should be selected based on the child's age and level of development, and that they should be administered appropriately to obtain an accurate assessment of pain. Therefore, it is important that healthcare professionals are trained in the use of these tools and ensure that they are used effectively to ensure the best possible pain management in children.

7. Conclusion

Pain is a subjective experience that can have a significant impact on the quality of life of children and adolescents. Therefore, it is critical to properly recognize, assess, and treat pain in this population. There are various treatment options available, including pharmacological pain relievers, psychological therapies, and less invasive surgical techniques. In addition, it is important to use pain assessment tools appropriate to the child's age and developmental level such as validated pain scales. The implementation of multidisciplinary strategies that address pain comprehensively can significantly improve pain management in children and adolescents.

Postoperative pain is a common consequence of pediatric surgery, but it can be effectively treated. It is important that parents and medical personnel work together to identify and treat pediatric postoperative pain and take steps to prevent its occurrence whenever possible. By doing so, patient discomfort can be minimized and a faster and more complete recovery promoted.

Pediatric pain medicine is a constantly evolving field, with multiple strategies and tools available to address pain in children and adolescents. Research has shown that proper pain management in children not only improves a patient's quality of life but can also reduce recovery time and length of hospital stay. In addition, a multidisciplinary approach and an individualized approach are essential to effectively treat pain in children. Less invasive anesthetic and surgical techniques, as well as anesthetic adjuvants, may be beneficial in managing postoperative pain in children. Relaxation methods, psychological therapies, and distraction strategies have also been shown to be effective in reducing preoperative anxiety and stress.

Finally, adequate assessment of pain in children is essential to achieve effective management. Pain measurement scales are an important tool and must be used regularly to identify pain and guide its treatment, so pain management in pediatrics is a crucial aspect of pediatric patient care and should continue to be investigated new strategies and tools to improve their treatment and relieve pain in children.

Author details

Alejandro Escalona-Espinosa[1*], Kelly Maldonado-Sánchez[2], Enrique Pazos-Alvarado[3], Pedro Castañeda[4], Rosina Alcaraz-Ramos[5], David Aguilar-Romero[6] and Keisuke Lira-Hernandez[7]

1 Hospital Español, CDMX, México

2 Hospital Infantil de México “Federico Gómez”, México

3 Hospital Infantil Privado “Star Médica,” México

4 Department of Pediatric Anesthesia and Pain Medicine, Hospital Infantil de México “Federico Gómez”, México

5 Hospital Infantil Tamaulipas, México

6 Hospital Ángeles Chihuahua, México

7 Hospital Español, Mexico

*Address all correspondence to: anestesiapediatrica@hotmail.com

References

[1] Pancekauskaitė G, Jankauskaitė L. Paediatric pain medicine: Pain differences, recognition and coping acute procedural pain in Paediatric emergency room. Medicina (B Aires). 2018;**54**(6):94

[2] Makhlouf MM, Garibay ER, Jenkins BN, Kain ZN, Fortier MA. Postoperative pain: Factors and tools to improve pain management in children. Pain Management. 2019;**9**(4):389-397

[3] Aldamluji N, Burgess A, Pogatzki-Zahn E, Raeder J, Beloeil H, Albrecht E, et al. PROSPECT guideline for tonsillectomy: Systematic review and procedure-specific postoperative pain management recommendations. Anaesthesia. 2021;**76**(7):947-961

[4] Chen Y-YK, Boden KA, Schreiber KL. The role of regional anaesthesia and multimodal analgesia in the prevention of chronic postoperative pain: A narrative review. Anaesthesia. 2021;**76**(S1):8-17

[5] Metz AK, Tomasevich KM, Froerer DL, Rosenthal RM, Featherall J, Aoki SK. Postoperative pain medication utilization in pediatric patients undergoing sports Orthopaedic surgery: Characterizing patient usage patterns and opioid retention. JAAOS: Global Research and Reviews. 2022;**6**(10):1-6

[6] Jones K, Engler L, Fonte E, Farid I, Bigham MT. Opioid reduction through postoperative pain Management in Pediatric Orthopedic Surgery. Pediatrics. 2021;**148**(6):e2020001487

[7] Aubrun F, Nouette-Gaulain K, Fletcher D, Belbachir A, Beloeil H, Carles M, et al. Revision of expert panel's guidelines on postoperative pain management. Anaesthesia, Critical Care & Pain Medicine. 2019;**38**(4):405-411

[8] Eldawlatly A. Bariatric anesthesia ladder. Saudi Journal of Anaesthesia. 2015;**9**(2):115

[9] Manworren RCB, Stinson J. Pediatric pain measurement, assessment, and evaluation. Seminars in Pediatric Neurology. 2016;**23**(3):189-200

[10] Fisher E, Law E, Dudeney J, Palermo TM, Stewart G, Eccleston C. Psychological therapies for the management of chronic and recurrent pain in children and adolescents. Cochrane Database of Systematic Reviews. 2014;**5**:CD003968

[11] Yang J, Zhang JW. Review of benefits and adverse effects of the most commonly used local anesthetic adjuvants in peripheral nerve blocks. Journal of Physiology and Pharmacology. 2022;**73**(3):337-346

[12] Meletti DP, Meletti JFA, Camargo RPS, Silva LM, Módolo NSP. Psychological preparation reduces preoperative anxiety in children. Randomized and double-blind trial. Journal of Pediatrics (Rio J). 2019;**95**(5):545-551

[13] Zieliński J, Morawska-Kochman M, Zatoński T. Pain assessment and management in children in the postoperative period: A review of the most commonly used postoperative pain assessment tools, new diagnostic methods and the latest guidelines for postoperative pain therapy in children. Advances in Clinical and Experimental Medicine. 2020;**29**(3):365-374

Chapter 7

Multimodal Pain Management in Extremely Low Birth Weight Neonates after Major Abdominal Surgery

Hana Jancova and Pavla Pokorna

Abstract

Limited data are available in the literature on multimodal pain management in extremely low birth weight (ELBW) neonates. This chapter aimed to summarize current knowledge about the effects of analgesics and sedatives (paracetamol, opioids, benzodiazepines and anaesthetics) on postoperative pain management ($\leq$ 48 hours after surgery). The primary endpoints of postoperative pain management were searched using validated pain assessment instruments, such as pain intensity, excessive sedation, drug consumption or adequate rescue medication. The secondary endpoints are the safety parameters of the drugs used, while the determinants of short/long-term outcome (duration of mechanical ventilation, intraventricular haemorrhage—IVH, periventricular leukomalacia—PVL, postnatal growth restriction, stage of chronic lung disease—CLD or neurodevelopmental outcome according to the Bayley-II Scale of Infant Development at 18–24 months or developmental equivalents at early-school age) were assessed as tertiary endpoints. Additionally, one of the most important key elements of clinical science is known as clinical research study validation, including specific tools and techniques within the validation processes. This chapter focuses on postoperative multimodal pain management, including the implementation of pain assessment tools and analgesic and sedative dosing regimens needed to achieve the efficacy and safety goals of an optimal pain profile in ELBW neonates; only proven non-pharmacological procedures are not included.

Keywords: extremely low birth weight neonates, postoperative pain, COMFORTneo score, paracetamol, opioid consumption

1. Introduction

Optimal pain management is an essential requirement of the daily clinical practice of a sick neonate and one of the indicators of quality-of-life care. Records of the experience of pain and its short-term and long-term consequences for the immature organism have been increasing in the recent decades, as well as warnings of the

IntechOpen

adverse effects of analgesics [1, 2]. A multimodal approach based on the multimodal concept of pain assessment can help to objectivate the diagnosis of pain in patients who are immature or who do not display pain due to severe illness. However, in non-verbal immature individuals, assessing pain or differentiating pain from discomfort is difficult and requires a specific approach and research into new diagnostic methods. The standard in clinical practice is evaluated scales mostly based on behavioural and physiological responses to pain. There are more than 65 assessment scales for childhood, but only a third of them are also validated for immature neonates, and significantly less for extremely low birth weight neonates (ELBW) after major abdominal surgery in particular [3]. Moreover, the choice of pain assessment tools varies among neonatal intensive care units (NICU) and countries as described, for example, in premature neonates treated for necrotizing enterocolitis (NEC) [4]. However, not all of the listed pain scales are validated, particularly for postoperative pain in ELBW.

To achieve the best possible quality in using these scoring systems at individual workplaces, implementing "evidence-based" procedures is necessary, including education with regular evaluation of the reliability and consistency of the staff in the assessment of pain since these methods are largely subjective. Objective methods such as measurement of tissue oxygenation (NIRS-near-infrared spectroscopy), skin conductance (SCM-skin conductance measurement), electroencephalography (EEG), or measurement of cortisol concentration in saliva or adrenaline, noradrenaline and cortisol determination in the blood, and physiological functions are currently auxiliary or research methods [5].

2. Clinical endpoints in neonatal postoperative pain studies

In general, clinical endpoints of pain studies are recommended to demonstrate that the introduction of validated pain together with sedation instruments while adjusting the age-appropriate dosage of analgesics and sedative drugs according to postmenstrual age (PMA) or postnatal age (PNA), and body weight leads to the

Name and type of scale, author, year, study design	Aim of the study	Indicators	Population settings (GW, pain profile, number of patients and diagnoses)	Drug used/ reported	Commentary/ limitations on scale
Neonatal facial coding scoring (NFCS), behavioural scale by *Peters et al., 2003* (prospective observational study)	Validitaion of the NFCS for postoperative pain, exploration of whether the number of NFCS items could be reduced	Brow bulge, eye squeeze, open lips, mouth and tongue position and lips pursed	29 GW to 18 M, ventilated child, prolonged pain, postoperative pain, 37 patients with abdominal/ thoracic surgery	Morphine	NFCS was found as a reliable, feasible and valid tool for assessing postoperative pain. Limitation: reduction of the NFCS to 5 items increases the specificity for pain assessment without reducing the sensitivity and validity for detecting changes in pain.

Name and type of scale, author, year, study design	Aim of the study	Indicators	Population settings (GW, pain profile, number of patients and diagnoses)	Drug used/ reported	Commentary/ limitations on scale
Children's & Infants' Postoperative Pain Scale (CHIPPS), behavioural scale, by *Büttner et al., 2000* (comprehensive report of 7 prospective studies)	Determination of parameters suitable indicators for postoperative pain	Crying, facial expression, trunk posture, legs movements, restlessness	35 GW to 5Y; postoperative pain, 584 children 4238 observations, diagnoses not reported	Not reported	Compared to other assessment tools (CHEOPS, OPS, CRIES, TPPPS), the CHIPPS scale items are most suitable for neonates, infants and young children in the postoperative period.
Pain Assessment Tool (PAT), multidimensional scale by *O'Sullivan et al., 2016* (non-randomised observational single-unit study)	Evaluation of the psychometric properties and clinical utility of the COVERS and PAT scales in a neonatal unit	Posture/tone, cry, sleep, face expression, colour, respiration, HR, SpO2, BP, nurse perception	23 GW to 6 M, postoperative pain, prolonged pain, 80 neonates (6 underwent surgery), diagnoses not reported	Not reported	Both COVERS* and PAT scales were reliable measures of acute pain in neonates from 24 GW. Most of the 72 assessing nurses preferred the COVERS (52%) to the PAT (16%), and 32% had no preference. Limitation: a small number of operated patients.
Modified Postoperative Comfort Score (PCS), behavioural scale, *by Guinsburg et al., 1998*, (randomised, double-blind, controlled trial)	Responses of ventilated preterm neonates to a single dose of fentanyl using physiological, humoral and behavioural measures	Sleep, facial expression, sucking, agitation, tonus, toe and finger posture, consolability	29 to 32 GW, ventilated patients, prolonged pain, 22 preterm ventilated neonates, diagnoses not reported	Fentanyl	The study demonstrated a reduction in both PCS and NFCS scores after initiation of fentanyl in preterm neonates on mechanical ventilation.
CRIES Scale, multidimensional scale, *Krechel et al., 1995*, prospective observational pilot study	Initial testing of validity and reliability of the CRIES	Crying, oxygen requires, vital signs, expression, sleeplessness	32 GW to 1 M, postoperative pain, acute pain, 24 infants following surgery (insertion of VP shunt, thoracotomy)	Not reported	The cutoff of oxygenation measure between scores 1 or 2 is set at 30%. This is not a suitable item for preterm infants with RDS/CLD. Alternatively, it can be substituted for respiratory changes in immature patients.

Name and type of scale, author, year, study design	Aim of the study	Indicators	Population settings (GW, pain profile, number of patients and diagnoses)	Drug used/ reported	Commentary/ limitations on scale
Multidimensional Assessment of Pain Scale (MAPS), multidimensional scale, by *Ramelet et al., 2007,* (follow-up validation study)	Evaluation of the clinical validity and utility of the MAPS and its response to the effect of analgesics	Vital signs (HR or BP), breathing pattern, facial expressions, body movements, state of arousal	36 GW to 31 M, postoperative pain 19 postoperative critically ill children	Morphine	This study showed that MAPS like FLACC and VAS decreased similarly following rescue morphine. Limitation: internal consistency of MAPS would improve if the psychologic item was deleted.

GW—gestational week, M—month, HR—heart rate, BP—blood pressure, COVERS—crying, oxygen requirement, vital signs, expression, resting, signalling distress, RDS—respiratory distress syndrome, CLD—chronic lung disease, VP—ventriculoperitoneal shunt.

Table 1.
Studies that reported postoperative pain management in preterm neonates – the list of validated scales in postoperative pain profile.

achievement of goals in the paediatric population [6]. More recently, the Neonatal Face Coding Score (NFCS) [7], the Children's & Infants' Postoperative Pain Scale (CHIPPS) [8], the Pain Assessment Tool (PAT) [9], the Modified Postoperative Comfort Score (PCS) = Clinical Scoring System [10], the CRIES scale [11] and the Multidimensional Assessment of Pain Scale (MAPS) [12] were validated for the treatment of postoperative pain in preterm neonates, of which only the PAT scale for extremely low birth weight neonates (ELBW, less than 1000 g, less than 28 weeks of gestation), respectively (**Table 1**). Therefore, in the ELBW cohort, it is also recommended that pain management, including assessment, re-evaluation, prevention, and treatment of a given pain profile (postoperative pain lasting 0–48 hours after surgery) adopted from other preterm neonates, seems to be best described by clinical goals. Primary endpoints are efficacy parameters (excessive, optimal or failed management) as measured by a validated postoperative score (PAT) or some validation processes are needed to be implemented using the COMFORTneo scale or the Numerical Rating Scale (NRS) for a given pain profile, and the effect of paracetamol on opioid consumption during the first 48 hours after surgery also. Secondary endpoints are, for example, safety parameters of the analgesic drugs (e.g., paracetamol hepatotoxicity or bradycardia <80/min, and hypotension defined as mean blood pressure < 10th percentile for opioids). Tertiary endpoints are parameters of long-term morbidity (e.g., intraventricular haemorrhage—IVH, periventricular leukomalacia—PVL, the severity of chronic lung disease, postnatal restriction of growth, prolonged pulmonary ventilatory support, abdominal discomfort, enteral nutrition and breastfeeding, length of hospital stay, and mental and psychomotor development in 12–24 months or death), and more recently, the correlation between total cumulative opioid dose from birth to the period of developmental equivalent assessment of cognitive, language, motor and executive functions at early-school age or later (**Figure 1**) [13].

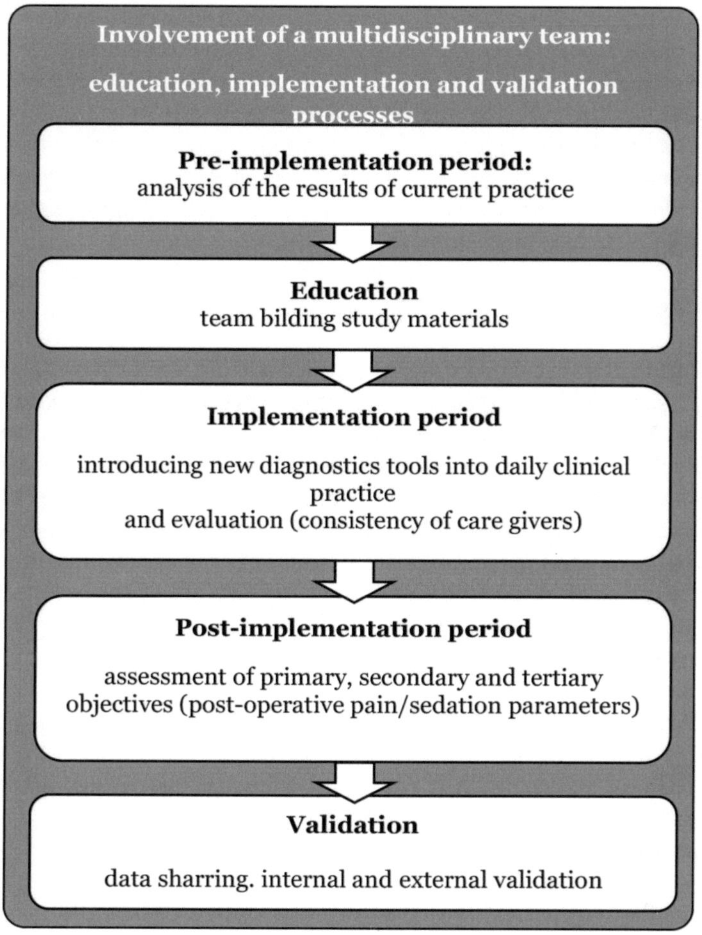

Figure 1.
Multimodal pain management in extremely low birth weight infants after major abdominal surgery and team involvement. Primary objectives are postoperative pain/sedation efficacy parameters (pain lasting 0–48 hours after surgery). Secondary objectives are safety parameters of the analgesics and sedative drugs used (pain lasting 0–48 hours after surgery). Tertiary objectives are parameters of long-term (monitoring parameters evaluated for 12–24 months) and early-school age (5 years of age).

3. Pain scales validated in ELBW population

3.1 Pain assessment tool (PAT)

The PAT scale is a scoring system developed and evaluated by Hodgkinson in 1994, originally in a group of 20 term neonates following surgery. The study found that PAT effectively quantified neonates' pain and reflected nurses' perceptions of it [14]. The scale incorporates both behavioural and physiological items and includes a score based on the caregiver's judgement to capture individual reactions and evaluations of the nurse who cared for the patient over time. The tool has ten parameters (see **Table 1**) that are scored on a scale of 0 to 2, with minimum and maximum scores of 0 and 20. Scores greater than 5 indicate some non-pharmacological methods to provide adequate comfort, and scores greater than 10 require adjustment of the analgesia. Later, Spence and O'Sullivan demonstrated that the PAT is a reliable and valid tool in various groups of NICU patients (both surgical and nonsurgical, preterm and term). The PAT is a clinician-friendly Pain Assessment Tool for all groups of critically ill infants in the NICU; moreover, according to the literature, it is the only scale validated for the postoperative pain profile in extremely low birth weight neonates [9, 15]. However, we find certain limitations in the small sample size of the studied surgical ELBW patients and in the possible impact of the variability of physiological thresholds across gestational/postmenstrual ages (e.g. chronic lung disease and oxygenation requirements).

3.2 COMFORTneo

In 2004, a modified COMFORT-behavioural scale (COMFORTneo) was created and validated in a population of preterm infants to provide the following definition: behavioural distress encompasses all behaviours of negative affect associated with pain, anxiety and fear. And distress may occur in the absence of pain [16]. The COMFORTneo scale consists of 6 behavioural items: alertness; calmness/agitation; muscle tone assessment by observation of movements of extremities, crying/respiratory response in ventilated patients, body movements and facial expressions. Total scores range from 6 to 30 (1 to 5 for each item) and the cutoff score reflecting pain/distress is ≥14. A score ≤ 9 reflects possible oversedation. Testing of internal consistency of the scale was good and concurrent validity with the NRS (Numeric rating scale) was adequate in terms of persistent or prolonged pain and sedation in neonates from the 23rd to 43rd weeks of gestational age. COMFORTneo scale and physiological measurements could be clinically useful pain instruments for the neonatal intensive care unit (NICU) environment and critically ill neonates in the postoperative period.

3.3 Numerical rating scale (NRS)

The NRS quantifies pain on a scale from 0 to 10 based on an individual patient's pain experience; the assessment of pain intensity is as follows: no pain = 0, mild pain = 1–3, moderate pain = 4–6, and severe pain ≥7. Various pictorial adaptations of the NRS mimicking facial expressions are used in young children. For non-verbal individuals, the quantification of pain rests in the hands of caregivers or parents according to the typical patient's pain behaviour. The tool's accuracy depends on the parents and nurse's ability to observe and describe the patient's response to pain in an individual way [17]. As some validation studies show, this simple tool is a good instrument to specify the nature of discomfort (pain or stress) as an additional tool along with validated behavioural and multidimensional scales in the population of preterm neonates [3]. The NRS is a useful instrument in the multimodal assessment of pain in premature neonates; moreover, the possibility of parental involvement in pain management improves current practice in NICUs.

4. Adjuvant objective methods in neonatal pain studies

4.1 Near-infrared spectroscopy (NIRS)

Cortical activity specifically associated with the affective component of nociception, i.e. with the negative emotional experience of pain (e.g. the area of the cingula, insula, prefrontal cortex), does not always have to be correlated with the discriminative-executive component, which we can assess from the behaviour of the neonates [18, 19]. NIRS is a non-invasive method of optical measurement of local changes in tissue oxygenation in real time. Roué described the most significant correlation between pain and changes in NIRS parameters in 113 full-term healthy neonates during venipuncture. The other measurements performed in this study (skin conductance, heart rate, cortisol in saliva) rather represented a prolonged stress reaction to pain [20]. Bartocci demonstrated primary and secondary somatosensory cortex activation after venipuncture in premature neonates (28-36th gestational weeks), with an intensity inversely proportional to gestational age [21]. Other CNS centres participating in the discriminative and affective components of nociception were also studied using this method. Yuan demonstrated a correlation between pain and NIRS changes in the prefrontal cortex during circumcision in healthy mature neonates [22]. NIRS is a non-invasive objective method that could most closely correlate with the cortical response to a painful stimulus.

4.2 Physiological functions

Heart and respiratory rate, SpO2 and blood pressure are measured continuously as a part of standard postoperative monitoring of vital functions. Physiological responses to pain stimuli and their correlations were described in multivariate analyses. In full-term infants, physiological measurements were not necessarily well-correlated with behavioural responses. A positive correlation was found between SpO2 and NIRS parameters (HbO2) [20]. Different findings were described in neonates between 28 and 36 weeks of gestation. Preterm infants were more likely to exhibit desaturation or apnoea in response to a painful or stressful stimulus [21]. Therefore, these different pain response profiles should be considered in future research.

4.3 Skin conductance measurement (SCM)

Changes in electrical skin conductance measured on the palmar side of the hands and soles appear suitable for objective pain evaluation [23, 24]. The activation of the sympathetic nervous system by painful stimuli leads to the activation of eccrine sweat glands and an increase in electrical skin conductivity. These changes could be detected in infants <28 + 0 of gestational age and seem to be able to differentiate between pain and discomfort [25]. Surprisingly, it seems that conductance parameters do not correlate with gestational age, and their changes have been described in neonates as early as 22 gestational weeks. The major limitation of the method is the inability to determine basal skin conductance in this population [26].

5. Pharmacological treatment in neonatal postoperative pain studies

Pharmacological treatment of pain together with sedation in the postoperative period is governed by international recommendations for the treatment of moderate to severe pain (postoperative pain profile lasting for 48 hours) for mechanically ventilated neonates, and a combination of systemic analgesics (opioids and non-opioids) and sedatives or regional anaesthesia (levobupivacaine) for some surgeries are selected [27]. Pharmacological treatment includes slow IV boluses, intermittent dosing or using continuous infusion with the commonly used opioid—morphine, and synthetic opioids—fentanyl, or sufentanil in some intensive care units, the effects of which are expressed as morphine potency. Therefore, morphine-equivalent doses are also calculated to achieve an analgesic effect, but the dosage will vary according to the postnatal age (PNA) of the neonate; for example, in neonates younger than 10 days, it is recommended to reduce the initial dose of morphine or sufentanil [28, 29]. More recently, alpha agonists (dexmedetomidine and clonidine) can also be considered, as well as intravenous paracetamol, recommended to be given to all patients regularly and in a dose corresponding to the postmenstrual age (PMA) with an initial loading dose and a maintenance dose (see paracetamol) [30, 31]. Adjusting the dosage of analgesics and sedative drugs is guided by the scale of pain and sedation and doses should be titrated to appropriate effects. In case of PAT score > 10 or COMFORTneo and NRS scores indicating discomfort (≥ 14 or more ≥4), the rate of opioid infusion is increased in individual steps by a certain percentage (%) up to the maximum age-appropriate dose to achieve the desired effect. As a rescue ("rescue") analgesic treatment in case of severe pain (i.e. PAT >10, COMFORTneo ≥ 22, NRS ≥ 7), a bolus of opioids or a second-choice drugs (e.g. ketamine, dexmedetomidine, clonidine or propofol) are used intravenously so that the target values of PAT (≤10), COMFORTneo (9–13) points and NRS (0–3 points) are achieved. On the contrary, for COMFORTneo scores corresponding to excessive sedation (<9) and NRS ≤3, the opioid infusion rate should be reduced, for example by a certain percentage (%) based on assessment. The analgesic/sedation concept in ELBW after abdominal surgery has its pharmacological aspects that strongly correlate with changes in drug disposition, which are the consequences of, for example, extreme immaturity, period of peri–/postoperative stress (metabolic, hormonal, etc.) related to abdominal causes of surgery (e.g. NEC, spontaneous intestinal perforation—SIP) or inflammation (changes in CYP 450 activity) or physiological changes in ventilation, circulation, renal and hepatic functions and as expected increased permeability of the blood-brain barrier to analgesics and sedatives in ELBW neonates. In this vulnerable population, therefore, measuring the effectiveness and safety of the drugs used is extremely important. In the following section, drugs are selected with a focus on drug characteristics, clinical indication, reported efficacy and safety and drug dosage in premature and ELBW neonates, respectively, after abdominal surgery. Complex therapy includes non-pharmacological interventions, sucrose, the most used intravenous analgosedative drugs (except ibuprofen), and significantly less used epidural analgesics; therefore, the knowledge about analgosedative use still missing in this population will be summarized.

5.1 Morphine

A natural opiate alkaloid with a rapid and prolonged peak onset of action (20 minutes after IV single injection) acting, for example 3–5 hours after IV single injection used in neonates for postoperative pain, for specific conditions such as necrotizing enterocolitis (NEC) and neonatal abstinence syndrome (NAS) [32, 33]. Pharmacodynamics is highly dependent on the dosage form and route of administration (epidural, intravenous, subcutaneous, intramuscular, oral or rectal) with a broad peak of onset of action after administration lasting between 20 and 90 min and a duration of 3–20 hours. However, ELBW neonates lack reports on efficacy and safety (e.g. evidence of benefits for poor neurologic outcomes) [34, 35]. Respiratory depression and hypotension have been described with continuous infusion. Therefore, lower doses are generally recommended in premature neonates. Dosing: analgesia [36, 37], 0.05–0.1 mg/kg/dose every 4–6-8 hours for intermittent dosing while for continuous IV infusion initial dose 0.01 mg/kg/dose is titrated to the maximum

0.03 mg/kg/hour (some authors suggested 0.015–0. 020 mg/kg/hour). Initial IV infusion rates of 0.010 mg/kg/hour are acceptable for neonates younger than 1 week. Neonates older than 1 week tolerate 0.015 mg/kg/hour, whereas older infants may tolerate 0.020–0.040 mg/kg/hour. Supplemental IV boluses of as much as 0.050 mg/kg may be administered for episodes of breakthrough pain in mechanically ventilated neonates who are receiving morphine by means of continuous infusion. For example, Kinderformularium recommends morphine dosing for preterm neonates < 37 weeks GA as an initial dose of 0.050–0.100 mg/kg followed by continuous infusion of 0.003–0.020 mg/kg/hour continuous infusion.

5.2 Fentanyl

Fentanyl is a synthetic effective opioid with high potency to morphine, a rapid-acting onset (peak onset 3–4 min after IV single injection) with medium-long duration (30 min after IV single injection) used for acute procedural, postoperative, and prolonged pain profile, and specific conditions (ECMO) in neonates. Adverse effects include apnoea, increased chest rigidity and respiratory depression that more often described when fentanyl is administered as an IV bolus of 0.001–0.002 mg/kg than when it is given as a continuous IV infusion of 0.001–0.002 mg/kg/hour while fentanyl causes less likely systemic hypotension than morphine. The first report of a cohort of very preterm neonates (23–30 gestational age) evaluated the association between cumulative neonatal exposure to fentanyl by neurodevelopmental and socioemotional outcomes in children at 5 years of age. However, according to the authors, the conclusions of this study were still ambiguous [38]. Dosing: analgesia [39], intermittent slow IV push 0.0005–0.003 mg/kg/dose, continuous infusion 0.0005–0.002 mg/kg/hour; sedation, slow IV push 0.001–0.004 mg/kg/dose may be repeated every 2–4 hours, continuous analgesia/sedation initial 0.001–0.002 mg/kg then 0.0005–0.001 mg/kg/hour. The mean required dose is 0.00064 mg/kg/hour <34 GA. During ECMO IV push 0.005–0.010 mg/kg and 0.001–0.005 (max 0.020) mg/kg/hour were reported due to known drug tolerance in this population. Additionally, the Kinderformularium database recommends fentanyl dosing for preterm neonates < 37 weeks GA: an initial dose of 0.0005–0.003 mg/kg followed by continuous infusion 0.005–0.003 mg/kg/hour continuous infusion.

5.3 Sufentanil

A synthetic, short-acting opioid agonist with a rapid onset of action (peak onset 5–6 min after IV single injection) and with a medium-long duration (30 min after IV single injection) more potent than fentanyl or morphine used for general and intraoperative anaesthesia, and analgesia/sedation in mechanically ventilated neonates and neonatal ECMO. Adverse effects are somewhat similar to those reported with fentanyl (bradycardia, hypotension, hypertension, cardiac arrhythmia, CNS depression, respiratory depression, chest wall rigidity, seizures and burst-suppression EEG pattern). Sufentanyl doses are not validated for premature neonates. Dosing: analgesia/sedation, in mechanically ventilated premature neonates 26–34 weeks IV loading dose 0.0005 mg/kg over 10 minutes followed by 0.002 mg/kg/hour continuous infusion [40], or in ventilated full-term neonates, sufentanil LD of 0.002 mg/kg and MD of 0.00029 mg/kg/hour was reported, but dosage regimen was recommended to be verified in clinical trials for analgesia in full-term neonates [41]. A 0.0005 mg/kg IV bolus and a continuous infusion of 0.0002 mg/kg/hour for 24 hours have been recommended for postoperative anaesthesia (Anand 1992). The Kinderformularium database recommends the dosage of sufentanil for young infants and children (from 1 month to 18 years)—an initial dose of 0.0002—0.0005 mg/kg (maximum 0.001 mg/kg) and a loading dose (LD) in ventilated patients: 0. 0003–0.002 mg/kg/dose slowly IV over 30 seconds. If necessary, additional doses of 0.0001–0.001 mg/kg/dose can be given up to a maximum (cumulative) dose of 0.005 mg/kg in major procedures [42].

5.4 Paracetamol

Paracetamol (acetaminophen) is a non-opioid drug commonly used drug to treat mild to moderate pain management (peak onset for analgesia from 5 to 10 min to 1 hour after IV single injection) and fever (peak onset antipyretic effect within 30 min after IV single infection) and pain profile with duration (4–6 hours for analgesia). It is successfully used for postoperative pain or as "rescue" treatment post-operatively, as reported in ELBW, and additionally, for narcotic and morphine-sparing effect, respectively [43]. At the same time, the administration of paracetamol only for procedural indications in neonates is under discussion [44]. Paracetamol is recommended for ELBW neonates intravenously post-operatively on a regular schedule as a slow bolus injection over 15 minutes, although evidence of paracetamol dosing for pain relief is also known for oral and rectal administration in younger neonates than 32 weeks of postmenstrual age (PMA). Concerns about adverse effects are justified (circulatory, hepatic, renal, respiratory, etc.), and dosing must be adjusted to the appropriate age of the neonate even though the production of hepatotoxic metabolites is lower due to reduced CYP450 activity [45]. Dosing: the loading dose of paracetamol for premature neonates is 20 mg/kg, and the maintenance dose (MD) is based on PMA: in neonates less than 32 weeks (PMA), the maintenance dose will be 7.5 mg/kg every 8 hours, in neonates ≥32 weeks of PMA 10 mg/kg every 8 hours [31]. Similarly, the Kinderformularium database recommends paracetamol dosing for premature neonates PMA < 32 weeks as a starting dose: 12 mg/kg/dose, once, and MD as 24 mg/kg/day in 4 doses intravenously [42].

5.5 Midazolam

Midazolam is, among other sedative drugs, still commonly used benzodiazepine with rapid onset action (within 1–5 min after IV single injection, maximum 5–7 min) and short duration (20-30 min after IV single injection) and widely used for sedative (acute/prolonged), anxiolytic and anticonvulsive effects and amnesia before induction of anaesthesia and procedural sedation used as intermittent dosing or continuous IV infusion. Adverse effects include cardiovascular (hypotension), seizure like-activity, myoclonic jerks in preterm neonates, nystagmus, agitation or bronchospasm. Dosing: sedation IV 0.05–0.15 mg/kg may be repeated every 2–4 hours, continuous IV infusion 0.01 to 0.06 mg /kg/hour, and the dose should be titrated to achieve the desired effect [46]. The Kinderformularium database recommends midazolam dosing for preterm neonates < 32 weeks GA: initial dose up to 8 weeks postnatal age (PNA) is 0.05 mg/kg/dose over 30 minutes to avoid the risk of hypotension if given more rapidly, and MD: 0.03 – 0.1 mg/kg/hour, continuous infusion [42].

5.6 Dexmedetomidine

An alfa (α-2) adrenergic agonist with rapid onset action (its onset of action is less than 5 minutes, and the peak effect occurs within 15 minutes) used for sedation, reversible hypnotic effect and added on analgesia profile for procedural sedation and is increasingly used post-operatively in neonates. The various reported side effects are hypotension, hypertension, nausea, vomiting, bradycardia, atrial fibrillation, and pyrexia, but no respiratory depression effects and less anaesthetics and fentanyl consumption were reported in some patient cohorts after abdominal surgery treated with dexmedetomidine perioperatively [47]. Dosing: initial bolus IV 0.00005–0.001 mg/kg over 10 min and continuous infusion 0.0002–0.0008 mg/kg/hour (max. 0.0012 mg/kg/hour). For example, the Kinderformularium database recommends dexmedetomidine dosing for preterm neonates < 37 weeks GA: LD 0.0002–0.0003 mg/kg/dose over 10 min and MD: 0.0002–0.0003 mg./kg/hour, continuous infusion dose based on effect and side effects. Max: 0.001 mg/kg/hour [42]. Use of LD (starting dose) depends on any concomitant use of other sedatives and the current and desired level of sedation.

5.7 Clonidine

An alfa (α-2)-adrenergic agonist with a rapid onset action and short duration (the peak action occurs in 10 minutes and lasts for 3–7 hours after IV single dose) that is used for its anxiolytic and sedative effects and safety profile (preventing respiratory depression or haemodynamic instability), treatment for NAS, although, withdrawal symptoms were reported similar but less likely to benzodiazepines and opioids [48]. There are various and unknown mechanisms related to its sedative and add-on analgesic effects. Dosing: 0.001–0.003 mg/kg over 10 min (max. 0.0012 mg/kg/day for intermittent dosing) or LD of 0.001 mg/kg over 10 min and 0.0005–0.001 mg/kg/hour [49, 50] in a term neonate. Also, the Kinderformularium database recommends clonidine dosing for term neonates only: LD 0.0005 mg/kg/hr., continuous infusion and MD up to a maximum of 0.003 mg/kg/hour, continuous infusion. If a rapid effect is desired, a loading dose of 0.001 mg/kg can be given in 15 minutes. Clonidine is reported to have a risk of rebound phenomenon after its discontinuation, so prevention of this phenomenon is recommended by slow weaning.

5.8 Ketamine

A general anaesthetic drug with a direct action on the cortex and limbic system with a rapid onset of action (within 30 seconds after IV injection), peak onset of action (5–6 min), and a medium-long duration following the IV single dose (5–10 minutes for anaesthesia) or over 15–30 min for analgesia after IM administration. Adverse effects are described among others (arrhythmias, bradycardia, tachycardia, hyper/hypotension, increased salivation, vomiting, tonic-clonic movements, airway obstructions, respiratory depression and hallucinations, etc., difficult to objectify in ELBW neonates) [51]. Dosing: LD 0.5–1.0 mg/kg (maximum 2 mg/kg) while using more smaller doses followed by IV continuous infusion 0.25 mg/kg/hour is more recently recommended [27] for a term neonate. The Kinderformularium doses are LD at induction of anaesthesia: 0.5–1 mg/kg/dose once and MD 0.5–3 mg/kg/hour continuous infusion [42]. Alternative: intermittent administration: 0.25–0.5 mg/kg/dose every 10–15 minutes [52].

5.9 Chloral hydrate

A hypnotic and sedative with CNS depressant properties similar to barbiturates. The onset of action is 10–20 minutes, peak effect within 30–60 min, and duration 4–8 hours. Adverse effects are described as CNS symptoms (paradoxical excitement),

EEG is not influenced, withdrawal syndrome is known for its prolonged use, and warnings are reported in the paediatric population [53–55]. It is used orally and rectally in neonates and is common for procedural sedation. The risk of accumulation is known after 3 days in preterm and 7 days in term neonates, and hypoxia may occur within 24 hours of administration in some reports. Dosing: 25–75 mg/kg max. á 12 h is administered orally/rectally in full-term neonates only 30 mg/kg/dose, once, and if necessary, repeat after 30 minutes with 15–30 mg/kg/dose [56, 57].

5.10 Propofol

Propofol (2,6-diisopropylphenol) is an anaesthetic drug with a fast onset of action (within 30 seconds) after IV injection and short-term anaesthetic effect (3–10 min) depending on the dose, infusion rate and duration of administration in mechanically ventilated neonates. Propofol is primarily used for induction/maintenance anaesthesia, acute/procedural sedation (e.g. endotracheal intubation), secondary to the treatment of seizures. However, side effects were described, including cardiovascular (dose-dependent profound and prolonged hypotension) in preterm neonates (25.8–31.7 gestational weeks) treated with or without hemodynamic instability and/or NEC if propofol was used as a premedication for sedation at intubation, then metabolic (hypertriglyceridemia), respiratory (apnoea) and life-threatening episodes were reported (propofol syndrome, CNS symptoms, etc.) [58, 59]. Dosing: for IV induction and the maintenance IV infusion with a starting dose of 1.0 and 1.5 mg/kg to a maximum of 3.5 mg/kg /hour [60].

6. Conclusion

In recent decades, many findings have been published on pain management in the neonatal population, increasingly in preterm neonates, but data are almost lacking for ELBW neonates and the relevant pain profile (postoperative pain) in this population. Except for clonidine, ketamine and chloral hydrate, drug doses have been published for some drugs (morphine, dexmedetomidine and fentanyl), especially in neonates below 37 weeks GA, and for paracetamol and midazolam in preterm neonates less than 32 weeks of PMA and GA respectively while insufficient data are available for fentanyl derivatives (sufentanil) in preterm neonates and especially in ELBW neonates. This period of life has specific pharmacological challenges due to extreme immaturity and unpredictable drug efficacy and safety, so any contribution of knowledge and established drug databases to optimize pain management in extremely low birth weight neonates using a multimodal approach to pain management is essential.

Acknowledgements

The authors would like to thank Prof. Dick Tibboel (Department of Paediatric Surgery, Erasmus Medical Center Sophia Children's Hospital, Rotterdam, The Netherlands) for retrieving the chapter.

Conflict of interest

The authors declare no conflict of interest.

Author details

Hana Jancova[1] and Pavla Pokorna[2,3,4,5]*

1 Division of Neonatology, Clinic of Gynaecology and Obstetrics, First Faculty of Medicine, Charles University and General University Hospital, Prague, Czech Republic

2 Department of Paediatrics and Inherited Metabolic Disorders, First Faculty of Medicine, Charles University and General University Hospital, Prague, Czech Republic

3 Department of Paediatric Surgery, Erasmus Medical Center Sophia Children's Hospital, Rotterdam, The Netherlands

4 Department of Physiology and Pharmacology, Karolinska Institutet and Karolinska University Hospital, Stockholm, Sweden

5 Institute of Pharmacology, First Faculty of Medicine, Charles University and General University Hospital, Prague, Czech Republic

*Address all correspondence to: pavla.pokorna@vfn.cz

References

[1] Simons SHP, van den Bosch GE, Tibboel D. Analgesic agents and sedatives. In: Aranda JV, editor. Neonatal and Pediatric Pharmacology, Therapeutic Principles in Practice. 5th ed. Philadelphia: Lippincott Williams & Wilkins; 2021. p. 972

[2] McPherson C, Miller SP, El-Dib M, Massaro AN, Inder TE. The influence of pain, agitation, and their management on the immature brain. Pediatric Research. 2020;**88**(2):168-175. DOI: 10.1038/s41390-019-0744-6

[3] Giordano V et al. Pain and sedation scales for neonatal and Pediatric patients in a preverbal stage of development: A systematic review. JAMA Pediatrics. 2019;**173**(12):1186-1197. DOI: 10.1001/jamapediatrics.2019.3351

[4] Barge JA et al. Current pain management practices for preterm infants with necrotizing enterocolitis: A European survey. Pediatric Research. 2023;**2023**. DOI: 10.1038/s41390-023-02508-2. PMID: 36828969

[5] Simons SHP et al. Randomised controlled trial evaluating effects of morphine on plasma adrenaline/noradrenaline concentrations in newborns. Archives of Disease in Childhood. Fetal and Neonatal Edition. 2005;**90**(1):36-41. DOI: 10.1136/adc.2003.046425

[6] Van Dijk M, Ceelie I, Tibboel D. Endpoints in pediatric pain studies. European Journal of Clinical Pharmacology. 2011;**67**(SUPPL. 1):61-66. DOI: 10.1007/s00228-010-0947-6

[7] Peters JWB et al. Neonatal facial coding system for assessing postoperative pain in infants: Item reduction is valid and feasible. The Clinical Journal of Pain. 2003;**19**(6):353-363. DOI: 10.1097/00002508-200311000-00003

[8] Büttner W, Finke W. Analysis of behavioural and physiological parameters for the assessment of postoperative analgesic demand in newborns, infants and young children: A comprehensive report on seven consecutive studies. Paediatric Anaesthesia. 2000;**10**(3):303-318. DOI: 10.1046/j.1460-9592.2000.00530.x

[9] O'Sullivan AT, Rowley S, Ellis S, Faasse K, Petrie KJ. The validity and clinical utility of the COVERS scale and pain assessment tool for assessing pain in neonates admitted to an intensive care unit. The Clinical Journal of Pain. 2016;**32**(1):51-57. DOI: 10.1097/AJP.0000000000000228

[10] Guinsburg R, Kopelman BI, Anand KJS, De Almeida MFB, Peres CDA, Miyoshi MH. Physiological, hormonal, and behavioral responses to a single fentanyl dose in intubated and ventilated preterm neonates. The Journal of Pediatrics. 1998;**132**(6):954-959. DOI: 10.1016/S0022-3476(98)70390-7

[11] Krechel SW, Bildner J. CRIES: A new neonatal postoperative pain measurement score. Initial testing of validity and reliabilityTitle. Pediatric Anesthesia. 1995;**5**(1):53-61. DOI: 10.1111/j.1460-9592.1995.tb00242.x

[12] Ramelet AS, Rees NW, McDonald S, Bulsara MK, Huijer Abu-Saad H. Clinical validation of the multidimensional assessment of pain scale. Paediatric Anaesthesia. 2007;**17**(12):1156-1165. DOI: 10.1111/j.1460-9592.2007.02325.x

[13] Van Den Bosch GE et al. Prematurity, opioid exposure and neonatal pain: Do they affect the developing brain? Neonatology. 2015;**108**(1):8-15. DOI: 10.1159/000376566

[14] Hodgkinson K, Bear M, Thorn J, Van Blaricum S. Measuring pain in neonates: Evaluating an instrument and developing a common language. The Australian Journal of Advanced Nursing. 1994;**12**(1):17-22

[15] Spence K, Gillies D, Harrison D, Johnston L, Nagy S. A reliable pain assessment tool for clinical assessment in the neonatal intensive care unit. JOGNN - Journal of Obstetric, Gynecologic, and Neonatal Nursing. 2005;**34**(1):80-86. DOI: 10.1177/0884217504272810

[16] Van Dijk M et al. Taking up the challenge of measuring prolonged pain in (premature) neonates the COMFORTneo scale seems promising. The Clinical Journal of Pain. 2009;**25**(7):607-616. DOI: 10.1097/AJP.0b013e3181a5b52a

[17] Solodiuk J, Curley MAQ. Pain assessment in nonverbal children with severe cognitive impairments: The individualized numeric rating scale (INRS). Journal of Pediatric Nursing. 2003;**18**(4):295-299. DOI: 10.1053/S0882-5963(03)00090-3

[18] Slater R, Cantarella A, Franck L, Meek J, Fitzgerald M. How well do clinical pain assessment tools reflect pain in infants? PLoS Medicine. 2008;**5**(6):0928-0933. DOI: 10.1371/journal.pmed.0050129

[19] Benoit B, Martin-Misener R, Newman A, Latimer M, Campbell-Yeo M. Neurophysiological assessment of acute pain in infants: A scoping review of research methods. Acta Paediatrics. 2017;**106**(7):1053-1066. DOI: 10.1111/apa.13839

[20] Roué JM, Rioualen S, Gendras J, Misery L, Gouillou M, Sizun J. Multi-modal pain assessment: Are near-infrared spectroscopy, skin conductance, salivary cortisol, physiologic parameters, and neonatal facial coding system interrelated during venepuncture in healthy, term neonates? Journal of Pain Research. 2018;**11**:2257-2267. DOI: 10.2147/JPR.S165810

[21] Bartocci M, Bergqvist LL, Lagercrantz H, Anand KJS. Pain activates cortical areas in the preterm newborn brain. Pain. 2006;**122**(1-2):109-117. DOI: 10.1016/j.pain.2006.01.015

[22] Yuan I et al. Functional near-infrared spectroscopy to assess pain in neonatal circumcisions. Paediatric Anaesthesia. 2022;**32**(3):404-412. DOI: 10.1111/pan.14326

[23] Walas W et al. Skin conductance measurement for the assessment of analgosedation adequacy in infants treated with mechanical ventilation: A multicenter pilot study. Advances in Clinical and Experimental Medicine. 2020;**29**(9). DOI: 10.17219/ACEM/126286

[24] Walas W, Halaba ZP, Szczapa T, Latka-grot J, Davis JM. Procedural pain assessment in infants without Analgosedation: Comparison of Newborn infant parasympathetic evaluation and skin conductance activity - A Pilot Study. Frontiers in Pediatrics. 2022;**9**(January):1-6. DOI: 10.3389/fped.2021.746504

[25] Munsters J, Wallström L, Ågren J, Norsted T, Sindelar R. Skin conductance measurements as pain assessment in newborn infants born at 22-27weeks gestational age at different postnatal age. Early Human Development. 2012;**88**(1):21-26. DOI: 10.1016/j.earlhumdev.2011.06.010

[26] Macko J, Moravcikova D, Kantor L, Kotikova M, Humpolicek P. Skin conductance as a marker of pain in infants of different gestational age. Biomedical Paper. 2014;**158**(4):591-595. DOI: 10.5507/bp.2013.066

[27] Allegaert K, van den Anker J. Sedation in the neonatal intensive care unit: International practice. In: Mason KP, editor. Pediatric Sedation outside of the Operating Room. Cham: Springer International Publishing; 2021. pp. 305-343. DOI: 10.1007/978-3-030-58406-1_18

[28] Krekels EHJ et al. Evidence-based morphine dosing for postoperative neonates and infants. Clinical Pharmacokinetics. 2014;**53**(6):553-563. DOI: 10.1007/s40262-014-0135-4

[29] Soreze Y et al. Reduced Sufentanil doses are effective for postoperative analgesia after ductal closure in extremely premature infants: A 10 years retrospective cohort study. The Clinical Journal of Pain. 2017;**33**(12):1109-1116. DOI: 10.1097/AJP.0000000000000487

[30] Allegaert K et al. Intravenous paracetamol (propacetamol) pharmacokinetics in term and preterm neonates. European Journal of Clinical Pharmacology. 2004;**60**(3):191-197. DOI: 10.1007/s00228-004-0756-x

[31] Allegaert K, Palmer GM, Anderson BJ. The pharmacokinetics of intravenous paracetamol in neonates: Size matters most. Archives of Disease in Childhood. 2011;**96**(6):575-580. DOI: 10.1136/adc.2010.204552

[32] ten Barge JA, Vermeulen MJ, Simons SHP, van den Bosch GE. Pain management for necrotizing enterocolitis: Getting the balance right. Pediatric Research. 2022;**2021**:1-9. DOI: 10.1038/s41390-022-01968-2

[33] Siu A, Robinson CA. Neonatal abstinence syndrome: Essentials for the practitioner. Journal of Pediatric Pharmacology and Therapeutics. 2014;**19**(3):147-155. DOI: 10.5863/1551-6776-19.3.147

[34] Simons S et al. Routine morphine infusion in preterm. JAMA. 2003;**290**(18):2419-2427. DOI: 10.1001/jama.290.18.2419

[35] Anand KJS et al. Morphine pharmacokinetics and pharmacodynamics in preterm and term neonates: Secondary results from the NEOPAIN trial. British Journal of Anaesthesia. 2008;**101**(5):680-689. DOI: 10.1093/bja/aen248

[36] Anand KJS. Opioid tolerance in neonates: A state-of-the-art review. Paediatric Anaesthesia. 2001;**11**(5):511-521. DOI: 10.1046/j.1460-9592.2001.00764.x

[37] Hegenbarth MA et al. Preparing for pediatric emergencies: Drugs to consider. Pediatrics. 2008;**121**(2):433-443. DOI: 10.1542/peds.2007-3284

[38] Mills KP, Lean RE, Smyser CD, Inder T, Rogers C, McPherson CC. Fentanyl exposure in preterm infants: Five-year neurodevelopmental and socioemotional assessment. Frontier in Pain Research. 2022;**3**(March):1-9. DOI: 10.3389/fpain.2022.836705

[39] Anand KJS et al. Consensus statement for the prevention and management of pain in the newborn. Archives of Pediatrics & Adolescent Medicine. 2001;**155**(2):173-180. DOI: 10.1001/archpedi.155.2.173

[40] Nguyen S, Vecchierini MF, Debillon T, Péréon Y. Effects of sufentanil on electroencephalogram in very and extremely preterm neonates. Pediatrics.

2003;**111**(1):123-128. DOI: 10.1542/peds.111.1.123

[41] Pokorná P, Šíma M, Koch B, Tibboel D, Slanař O. Sufentanil disposition and pharmacokinetic model-based dosage regimen for Sufentanil in ventilated full-term neonates. Pharmacology. 2021;**106**(7-8):384-389. DOI: 10.1159/000515787

[42] Kinderformularium. [Internet]. [cited 2023 Apr 4]. Available from: https://www.kinderformularium.nl/

[43] Cihlarova H, Bencova L, Zlatohlavkova B, Allegaert K, Pokorna P. Rescue paracetamol in postoperative pain management in extremely low birth weight neonates following abdominal surgery: A single unit retrospective study. Frontiers in Pediatrics. 2022;**10**(June):1-8. DOI: 10.3389/fped.2022.895040

[44] Allegaert K. A critical review on the relevance of paracetamol for procedural pain management in neonates. Frontiers in Pediatrics. 2020;**8**(89). DOI: 10.3389/fped.2020.00089

[45] Lauterburg JR, Vaishnav BH, Stillwell Y, Mitchell WG. The effects of age and glutathione depletion on hepatic glutathione turnover in vivo determined by acetaminophen probe analysis. The Journal of Pharmacology and Experimental Therapeutics. 1980;**213**(1):54-58

[46] Völler S et al. Recently registered midazolam doses for preterm neonates do not Lead to equal exposure: A population pharmacokinetic model. Journal of Clinical Pharmacology. 2019;**59**(10):1300-1308. DOI: 10.1002/jcph.1429

[47] Weerink MAS, Struys MMRF, HannivoortLN,BarendsCRM,AbsalomAR, Colin P. Clinical pharmacokinetics and pharmacodynamics of Dexmedetomidine. Clinical Pharmacokinetics. 2017;**56**(8):893-913. DOI: 10.1007/s40262-017-0507-7

[48] R. Yasaei and A. Saadabadi, "Clonidine." StatPearls Publishing, Treasure Island (FL), 2022. Available: https://www.ncbi.nlm.nih.gov/books/NBK459124/ [Accessed: February 23, 2023]

[49] Ambrose C et al. Intravenous clonidine infusion in critically ill children: Dose-dependent sedative effects and cardiovascular stability. British Journal of Anaesthesia. 2000;**84**(6):794-796. DOI: 10.1093/oxfordjournals.bja.a013594

[50] Micormedex NeoFax Essentials. 2022. Available: https://www.micromedexsolutions.com [Accessed: February 24, 2023]

[51] Saarenmaa E, Neuvonen PJ, Huttunen P, Fellman V. Ketamine for procedural pain relief in newborn infants. Archives of Disease in Childhood. 2001;**85**(1):53-56. DOI: 10.1136/fn.85.1.f53

[52] Kinderformularium: Esketamine. https://www.kinderformularium.nl/geneesmiddel/137/esketamine [Accessed: February 27, 2023]

[53] Ikbal M, Tastekin A, Dogan H, Pirim I, Ors R. The assessment of genotoxic effects in lymphocyte cultures of infants treated with chloral hydrate. Mutational Research. 2004;**564**(2):159-164. DOI: 10.1016/j.mrgentox.2004.08.007

[54] Cruise S, Tam-Chan D, Harrison D, Johnston L. Prospective clinical audit of chloral hydrate administration practices in a neonatal unit. Journal of Paediatrics and Child

Health. 2012;**48**(11):1010-1015. DOI: 10.1111/j.1440-1754.2012.02586.x

[55] Hershenson M, Brouillette RT, Olsen E, Hunt CE. The effect of chloral hydrate on genioglossus and diaphragmatic activity. Pediatric Research. 1984;**18**(6):516-519. DOI: 10.1203/00006450-198406000-00006

[56] Finnemore A et al. Chloral hydrate sedation for magnetic resonance imaging in newborn infants. Paediatric Anaesthesia. 2014;**24**(2):190-195. DOI: 10.1111/pan.12264

[57] Allegaert K, Daniels H, Naulaers G, Tibboel D, Devlieger H. Pharmacodynamics of chloral hydrate in former preterm infants. European Journal of Pediatrics. 2005;**164**(7):403-407. DOI: 10.1007/s00431-005-1648-5

[58] Allegaert K et al. Inter-individual variability in propofol pharmacokinetics in preterm and term neonates. British Journal of Anaesthesia. 2007;**99**(6):864-870. DOI: 10.1093/bja/aem294

[59] Allegaert K, Peeters MY, Knibbe C. Propofol in (pre)term neonates: Consider the extensive interindividual variability in clearance within the neonatal population. Pediatric Anesthesia. 2011;**21**(2):174-175. DOI: 10.1111/j.1460-9592.2010.03482.x

[60] de Kort EHM, Twisk JWR, van Verlaat EPG, Reiss IKM, Simons SHP, van Weissenbruch MM. Propofol in neonates causes a dose-dependent profound and protracted decrease in blood pressure. Acta Paediatric. 2020;**109**(12):2539-2546. DOI: 10.1111/apa.15282

Chapter 8

Postoperative Sore Throat

Lorena Bobadilla Suárez, Ailyn Cendejas Schotman, Jonathan Jair Mendoza Reyes, Luisa Fernanda Castillo Dávila and Fernando Mondragón Rodríguez

Abstract

Postoperative sore throat is a common complaint amongst patients who have received general anesthesia and airway management. Several risk factors have been associated to the presence of postoperative sore throat as well as interventions aimed at reducing the incidence and intensity of the pain. The intensity of pain varies widely through populations and can be as insignificant as a complaint or negatively associated with the quality of care during a procedure. The length of duration can be from a few hours postoperatively up to a couple of days following the procedure and is also linked to some surgical related factors. To this day there is no consensus on the best way to prevent its appearance but understanding its pathophysiology as well as how our medical interventions can affect the patient's outcome is a step forward towards decreasing its significance in the postoperative setting.

Keywords: postoperative sore throat, hoarseness, postoperative pain, airway management complications, quality of care

1. Introduction

The incidence of postoperative sore throat (POST) varies depending on the source from 15 to 60%. POST is mainly caused due to the pressure that the airway device exerts on the respiratory mucosa. This pressure causes a reduction in blood flow through the small capillaries which can cause an anoxic-ischemic local reaction. The pressure and local inflammatory mediators can also activate local c fibers that signal pain. The airway devices are made of silicone and PVC which even when lubricated can adhere to the mucosa due to a normal reduction in local secretion of mucus secondary to the presence of a foreign body and cause trauma when removing the device. In long procedures, the slight movements of the device can cause chafing of the area, and local inflammation. The excessive manipulation of the airway in the presence of a difficult intubation or inadequate laryngeal mask airway (LMA) size causes edema that can further add to the inflammation and pain present in the postoperative period. It has been theorized that the passage of cold anesthetic and medicinal gases in the airway through the devices can also be a cause of airway irritation, similar to the use of supplemental oxygen through nasal tips, but more evidence is necessary to confirm this. It is evident that several factors add to the presence of inflammation and mucosa

IntechOpen

lesion which can be reduced by increasing awareness amongst anesthesiologists of its importance. In 2010, a bi-continental survey demonstrated that patient dissatisfaction is often due to postoperative nausea and vomiting (PONV) followed by POST [1]. This highlights the need for our attention to this symptom and maneuvers aimed towards preventing or reducing it.

2. Risk factors associated with POST

Risk factors have been largely identified in both patient specific details, as well as surgical and anesthetic related factors. It is important to identify the patients risk factors to plan accordingly and prevent this undesirable symptom when its presence is looming. Pain is a subjective feeling and therefore can be influenced by the patient's state of mind prior to the procedure. Anxious patients are more likely to refer POST as well as perceive a higher intensity of the pain. Sufficient information about what to expect upon anesthesia emersion is important to help the patient cope with these symptoms as they appear.

2.1 Age

There have been different results depending on the population studied and have found conflicting results. Some authors have found a higher incidence amongst young patients [2], and others claim the incidence is higher amongst geriatric patients [3]. It is well known that as we age, our nervous fibers become less sensitive to pain stimuli, so it is probable that the risk factor of old age is more associated to difficult airways that are common in geriatric patients, rather than old age itself.

2.2 Sex

Authors agree that female patients are more likely to report the presence of POST as well as a higher incidence of intense pain [1, 4, 5]. This is explained due to smaller airways in females in comparison to males which can translate to a tighter fit of the device in the airway.

2.3 Airway device

POST is present in higher proportion of patients in which endotracheal intubation was the airway management of choice compared to LMA [6, 7], and the incidence is even higher when and endobronchial tube is used [2, 8, 9]. POST can be reduced or even prevented in some cases with the use of a video laryngoscope [10], to reduce airway manipulation and number of intubation attempts.

2.4 Difficult airway

Patients with predicted difficult airways, are more likely to present POST due to the use of intubation stylets, multiple attempts for intubation or vocal cord lesion. This risk is even greater when the difficult airway is not predicted during preoperative evaluation due to an inefficient planning, which may result in even more airway manipulation, and a blood stained ETT is more probable upon extubation.

2.5 Endotracheal tube size

POST is importantly linked to the use of larger lumen endotracheal tubes (ETT). Many authors have found a lower incidence of POST when reducing the ETT size [2, 3, 5, 6] even by 0.5 mm. Traditionally, larger ETT were selected to reduce airflow resistance and provide better ventilation, but this intervention has little significance when the ventilation is transitory as is in a surgical procedure. The adequate size of ETT has not been determined to avoid adverse events regarding mechanical ventilation, but a simple reduction in 0.5 mm in the size normally selected in healthy patients seems to be a safe choice to reduce incidence of POST.

Nasotracheal intubation is also associated with higher incidence of POST due to manipulation of the airway, ETT size and blood stained ETT upon removal. Until now, the only maneuver that seems to reduce this risk when selecting nasotracheal intubation is the use of fiberscope for its insertion as opposed to manual insertion assisted by laryngoscopy and Magill clamps.

2.6 Cuff pressure

When using ETT or LMA, guidelines have always recommended the use of a manometer to maintain cuff pressure ETT between 20 and 30 cmH2O and to monitor every 30 minutes, or less if using nitrous oxide. Adequate control of intracuff pressure can help reduce the incidence of POST [11].

The objective in the case of LMA is to not exceed 60 cmH2O. On occasion, following the manufacturer's recommended fill volumes, pressures above 60 cmH2O can be obtained [12].

2.7 Muscle relaxants

The use of succinylcholine has been associated with the presence of POST [2] probable secondary to muscle fasciculations and intense potassium release that can add to the known POST risk factors.

In emergency settings, some medical professionals may choose to avoid muscle relaxants which can cause vocal cord lesions and elevate the risk for POST.

2.8 Anesthetic related factors

POST is usually present when the airway manipulation has been excessive. This can be associated with difficult airway, use of intubation stylets and use of direct laryngoscopy. Some authors have proposed that the expertise of the person who performs the laryngoscopy could be a factor leading to presence of POST, but there are conflicting results. What has been demonstrated is that a low time to secure the airway can drastically reduce the incidence of POST [5]. Blood stained ETT upon extubation has been linked to POST [9] which is expected since it is evidence of excessive airway manipulation or use of a large ETT.

2.9 Surgical related factors

Long procedures resulting in endotracheal intubation for 3 hours or more was highly associated to POST [3]. Gynecologic surgery has also been linked to higher incidence of POST that can probably be explained by the extreme Trendelenburg position required for many laparoscopic gynecologic procedures which elevate the pressure in the airway secondary to blood pooling in the upper body [9]. Head and neck surgery has also been linked to higher incidence of POST, particularly otorhinolaryngologic surgery.

3. Interventions for reducing incidence and intensity of POST

Interventions to reduce the incidence and/or severity of POST have been largely studied varying from nebulized corticosteroids or magnesium, licorice, or ketamine gargles, intracuff saline or lidocaine, and lidocaine or benzydamine spray on the outside of the airway device. Non-pharmacological interventions consist in avoiding large ETT and high-pressure cuffs as well as the use of a manometer to control the cuff pressure during the procedure. The use of video laryngoscopy can reduce the incidence of POST in difficult airways as it reduces the number of attempts to intubation and reduces airway manipulation, but the use of stylets has been associated with a higher incidence of POST and several video laryngoscopes need a specific stylet for the curvature of each device.

3.1 Lidocaine spray

Lidocaine spray has proved NOT to decrease the intensity or presence of POST and can even be linked to worse outcomes [13]. The lidocaine's vehicle creates a film over the mucosa and prevents normal secretion. This film then adheres to the mucosa and can cause lesion and irritation when the device is removed.

3.2 Intracuff lidocaine

Lidocaine can permeate through the cuff towards the area of contact due to the cuff's semipermeable nature. The lidocaine tends to diffuse towards the area with a lower concentration and attempts to achieve pH balance. Studies have shown that the diffusion is consequently facilitated if the lidocaine is alkalinized. Authors agree that a relation of 2% lidocaine 9 ml: sodium bicarbonate 7.5% 1 ml is an adequate solution for optimal diffusion [4]. Intracuff alkalinized lidocaine can reduce the incidence and severity of POST up to 50% [14, 15].

3.3 Benzydamine spray

Benzydamine spray on the outside of the device has been widely used with much better results that lidocaine spray, reducing the incidence of POST in comparison to placebo but has not been effective in concomitant use with intracuff lidocaine [4, 16].

3.4 NDMA antagonists

Magnesium has been shown to be more effective than ketamine to reduce the incidence and severity of POST [13, 17] but has little clinical use due to the difficulty for preoperative nebulization as well as the added costs in both public and private settings since the equipment for nebulization is not generally necessary in a healthy patient undergoing surgery.

3.5 Multimodal analgesia

With the advent of the opioid crisis across the globe, multimodal analgesia has become much more appreciated. Current recommendations include the use of opioids as rescue analgesics in the post-anesthesia care unit (PACU). Conventional analgesia generally includes a non-steroidal anti-inflammatory (NSAID) drug, paracetamol/acetaminophen, and a short life steroid. POST has been compared in patients who have received multimodal analgesia vs. single drug analgesia and have found a superiority of dexamethasone in combination with other analgesic drugs for the reduction in incidence and severity of POST [18, 19]. Opioid sparing anesthesia has also proven beneficial to reduce the incidence of POST, mainly secondary to the use of intravenous lidocaine, magnesium and/or dexmedetomidine in perfusion [19].

4. Conclusion

When patients present with more than one risk factor, we recommend interventions on behalf of the anesthesia providers to reduce the incidence and intensity of POST. In healthy patients, one may consider the use of a smaller ETT with the concomitant cuff pressure control with the use of a manometer. The use of benzydamine spray on the outside of the ETT or alkalinized lidocaine inside the cuff have proven to be effective and low-cost interventions which can reduce the intensity of POST. The use of multimodal analgesia has been recommended for a few years now as a staple for any anesthetic procedure and can be extremely beneficial for the prevention of POST. Intravenous lidocaine before suction and extubation can reduce the presence of coughing, and improve ETT tolerance upon emersion [20], given the patient has no contraindication for its use which is beyond the scope of this chapter.

Additionally, extubation parameters may contribute to POST, including but not limited to blood stained ETT, presence of blood during suctioning, coughing during emersion and delay to extubation once awake [21]. These factors are usually associated with those above mentioned as are difficult airway and excessive airway manipulation. These parameters can be modified or prevented in some cases with maneuvers such as use of multimodal anesthesia or lidocaine bolus to increase ETT tolerance upon emersion and suctioning.

POST is a very common complaint following anesthetic procedures and should not be overlooked.

Conflict of interest

The authors declare no conflict of interest.

Appendices and nomenclature

POST	postoperative sore throat
PONV	postoperative nausea and vomiting
LMA	laryngeal mask airway
ETT	Endotracheal tube
PACU	post-anesthesia care unit
NSAID	non-steroidal anti-inflammatory

Author details

Lorena Bobadilla Suárez[1*], Ailyn Cendejas Schotman[2], Jonathan Jair Mendoza Reyes[2], Luisa Fernanda Castillo Dávila[1] and Fernando Mondragón Rodríguez[3]

1 Department of Anesthesia, Hospital General de México, "Dr. Eduardo Liceaga", Mexico City, Mexico

2 Department of Anesthesia, Hospital Ángeles del Pedregal, Mexico City, Mexico

3 Department of Transplants, Hospital General de México, "Dr. Eduardo Liceaga", Mexico City, Mexico

*Address all correspondence to: dra.lorena.bobadilla@gmail.com

References

[1] Lehmann M, Monte K, Barach P, Kindler CH. Postoperative patient complaints: A prospective interview study of 12,276 patients. Journal of Clinical Anesthesia [Internet]. 2010;**22**(1):13-21

[2] El-Boghdadly K, Bailey CR, Wiles MD. Postoperative sore throat: A systematic review. Anaesthesia [Internet]. 2016;**71**(6):706-717

[3] Jiang J, Wang Z, Xu Q, Chen Q, Lu W. Development of a nomogram for prediction of postoperative sore throat in patients under general anaesthesia: A single-Centre, prospective, observational study. BMJ Open [Internet]. 2022;**12**(5):e059084

[4] Bobadilla SL, Gutiérrez S, Portela O. Comparison between postoperative sore throat in adults subjected to orotracheal intubation for elective surgery with the use of benzydamine, alkalinized lidocaine and placebo, alone or combined. Randomized clinical trial. Acta Medica [Internet]. 2021;**19**(1):89-91

[5] Mitobe Y, Yamaguchi Y, Baba Y, Yoshioka T, Nakagawa K, Itou T, et al. A literature review of factors related to postoperative sore throat. Journal of Clinical Medical Research [Internet]. 2022;**14**(2):88-94

[6] Xu R, Lian Y, Li WX. Airway complications during and after general anesthesia: A comparison, systematic review and meta-analysis of using flexible laryngeal mask airways and endotracheal tubes. PLoS One [Internet]. 2016;**11**(7):e0158137

[7] Scuderi PE. Postoperative sore throat: More answers than questions. Anesthesia and Analgesia [Internet]. 2010;**111**(4):831-832

[8] Park S-H, Han S-H, Do S-H, Kim J-W, Rhee K-Y, Kim J-H. Prophylactic dexamethasone decreases the incidence of sore throat and hoarseness after tracheal extubation with a double-lumen endobronchial tube. Anesthesia and Analgesia [Internet]. 2008;**107**(6):1814-1818

[9] Flexman AM, Duggan LV. Postoperative sore throat: Inevitable side effect or preventable nuisance? Canadian Journal of Anaesthesia [Internet]. 2019;**66**(9):1009-1013

[10] Lee JY, Hur HJ, Park HY, Jung WS, Kim J, Kwak HJ. Comparison between video-lighted stylet (Intular ScopeTM) and direct laryngoscope for endotracheal intubation in patients with normal airway. The Journal of International Medical Research [Internet]. 2020;**48**(11):030006052096953

[11] Liu J, Zhang X, Gong W, Li S, Wang F, Fu S, et al. Correlations between controlled endotracheal tube cuff pressure and postprocedural complications: A multicenter study. Anesthesia and Analgesia [Internet]. 2010;**111**(5):1133-1137

[12] Bick E, Bailes I, Patel A, Brain AI. Fewer sore throats and a better seal: Why routine manometry for laryngeal mask airways must become the standard of care. Anaesthesia [Internet]. 2014;**69**(12):1304-1308

[13] Wang G, Qi Y, Wu L, Jiang G. Comparative efficacy of 6 topical pharmacological agents for preventive interventions of postoperative sore throat after tracheal intubation: A systematic

review and network meta-analysis. Anesthesia and Analgesia [Internet]. 2021;**133**(1):58-67

[14] Estebe J-P, Gentili M, Le Corre P, Dollo G, Chevanne F, Ecoffey C. Alkalinization of intracuff lidocaine: Efficacy and safety. Anesthesia and Analgesia [Internet]. 2005;**101**(5):1536-1541

[15] Lam F, Lin Y-C, Tsai H-C, Chen T-L, Tam K-W, Chen C-Y. Effect of intracuff lidocaine on postoperative sore throat and the emergence phenomenon: A systematic review and meta-analysis of randomized controlled trials. PLoS One [Internet]. 2015;**10**(8):e0136184

[16] Kuriyama A, Aga M, Maeda H. Topical benzydamine hydrochloride for prevention of postoperative sore throat in adults undergoing tracheal intubation for elective surgery: A systematic review and meta-analysis. Anaesthesia [Internet]. 2018;**73**(7):889-900

[17] Mayhood J, Cress K. Effectiveness of ketamine gargle in reducing postoperative sore throat in patients undergoing airway instrumentation: A systematic review. JBI Database of Systematic Reviews and Implementation Reports [Internet]. 2015;**13**(9):244-278

[18] Jiang Y, Chen R, Xu S, Li J, Yu F, Kong L, et al. The impact of prophylactic dexamethasone on postoperative sore throat: An updated systematic review and meta-analysis. Journal of Pain Research [Internet]. 2018;**11**:2463-2475

[19] Yang SS, Wang N-N, Postonogova T, Yang GJ, McGillion M, Beique F, et al. Intravenous lidocaine to prevent postoperative airway complications in adults: A systematic review and meta-analysis. British Journal of Anaesthesia [Internet]. 2020;**124**(3):314-323

[20] Tanaka Y, Nakayama T, Nishimori M, Tsujimura Y, Kawaguchi M, Sato Y. Lidocaine for preventing postoperative sore throat. Cochrane Database of Systematic Reviews [Internet]. 2015;**14**(7):1-15

[21] Sakkanan NV, Elakkumanan LB. Extubation parameters and postoperative sore throat. Anesthesia and Analgesia [Internet]. 2020;**130**(2):e42-e43

Chapter 9

Non-Pharmacological Management of Acute Pain after Breast and Thoracic Surgery

Yetunde Oluwafunmilayo Tola, Ka Ming Chow, Wei Liang, Esther Ilesanmi, Oluwatosin Comfort Olarinde and Deborah Blessing Odejobi

Abstract

Pain after thoracic and breast surgery is a common phenomenon, and it is usually influenced by various factors including surgical, patient, and cultural factors. However, the pain that patients who have undergone breast or thoracic surgery experience has either been overlooked, undermanaged, or managed solely with pharmacotherapy by healthcare providers. This oftentimes result in impacting the patients' recovery process and even quality of life. Literature has identified that inadequate pain management after breast and thoracic surgery and the resultant side effects of pharmacological therapies can be reduced by including non-pharmacological interventions into patients' care plan. Some of the recommended interventions include music, massage, aromatherapy, cold therapy, meditation, acupuncture, and transcutaneous electrical nerve stimulation. Most of these non-pharmacological therapies are easy to use, promote patients' involvement in their own care, have no or minimal side effect, and are cost-effective. Therefore, it is essential for healthcare providers to include non-pharmacological pain management in the plan of care even before surgery.

Keywords: acute pain, non-pharmacological, management, breast surgery, thoracic surgery

1. Introduction

Postoperative pain is generally short term and acute in nature. It arises from injury of tissue which resulted from surgical procedures [1, 2]. Of all surgical procedures, thoracic and breast surgeries cause significant severe postoperative pain and suffering to patients [3]. For this reason, provision of adequate and effective postoperative pain relief is the paramount goal for thoracic and breast surgery patients during postoperative period. Inadequate pain management after surgery can be caused by several reasons including limited translation of current best available evidence to guide quality pain management in clinical praxis [4]. Standardised and streamlined pain management of patients who undergo these surgeries also requires knowledge and concept of evidence-based interventions to assure the quality and success of the management.

2. Postoperative pain after thoracic surgery

Thoracic surgery involves several pain sensitive structures with a number of pain transmission and perception; hence, patients are expected to experience severe pain within the first 72 hours after surgery [5]. Arising from surgical approaches and intraoperative manipulations of the thoracic structures, pain after thoracic surgery is commonly acute in nature with high severity in the immediate postoperative period [5]. Some of the descriptors used by patients to describe pain after thoracic surgery may be suggestive of mixed pain (acute pain and neuropathic pain), which when not adequately managed can result in chronic pain [6, 7].

Post-thoracic surgery pain has a complex mechanism that mostly occurs due to nociceptive and neuropathic signals that originate from somatic and visceral afferents [8]. Nociceptors are stimulated by the skin incision, muscle retraction, rib retraction, stretched ligaments, costochondral joint dislocation, and intercostal nerves injury [9–11].

Due to intra- and postoperative thoracic surgical approach and manipulation, noxious stimuli are transmitted by the intercostal nerve from the structures of the chest wall and pleura cavity to the nociceptive neurons in the central nervous system [8, 12]. The ipsilateral dorsal horn of the spinal cord (T4–T10) receives nociceptive somatic signals after a surgical trauma (incision, retraction, etc.) to the thoracic area [8, 11]. Then, the afferents are transmitted to the limbic system and somatosensory cortices through the contralateral anterolateral system.

Surgical manipulations of the structures of the chest including the pleura, diaphragm, or bronchi also initiate visceral stimuli. Nociceptive visceral afferents stimulated from tissue injury around bronchi and visceral pleura are transmitted by the vagus and phrenic nerves, the noxious stimuli arising from the diaphragmatic pleura are transmitted via the phrenic nerve, while mediastinum, lungs, and mediastinal pleura noxious stimuli are transmitted by the vagus nerve to the pain receptor [8]. Noxious stimuli resulting from surgical incision-induced tissue damage around the surgical sites are transmitted to the pain receptor in the central nervous system. These transmissions activate and sensitise nociceptor to develop an inflammatory response which further stimulates nociceptors and amplifies the transmission of pain, thereby increasing pain perception and hyperalgesia or increasing pain intensity at the surgical site [12].

Furthermore, noxious stimuli as afferent impulses resulting from visceral pleura irritation are referred to the ipsilateral shoulder by the phrenic nerves and become the major cause of ipsilateral shoulder pain after thoracic surgical procedures or post-thoracotomy shoulder pain [9–11]. Additionally, pain development is exaggerated by brachial plexus stretching and posterior thoracic ligaments distraction [11, 13]. Shoulder pain after thoracic surgery is often developed in the early stage or immediately after surgery lasting for a few days with usually moderate to severe intensity and mostly described by patients as an ache [14].

Compression and irritation of the intercostal nerves by chest tubes and surgical stripping or residual pleural blood may further activate inflammatory response [8, 9]. Consequently, inflammatory mediators (e.g. prostaglandins, histamine, bradykinin, and potassium) are released [8–11]. The release of prostaglandins, neurotrophins, and interleukins contributes to the activation of nociception and sensitisation [12].

Damage to nerves, most often the intercostal nerve injury resulting from mechanical damage, rib retractor, compression, or rib fractures as well as phrenic nerve irritation from chest tube placement has been reported in the literature as major contributors to neuropathic pain. Chest tubes after thoracic surgery also cause severe pain in cases where the tubes compress the intercostal nerves. In addition, the presence of sutures or wires passed around the ribs and closer to the neurovascular bundle may result in intercostal nerves damage, thus leading to neuropathic pain [11].

In a nutshell, for most patients undergoing thoracic surgery, there are several components and mechanisms that contribute to pain development. This may be a combination of acute, somatic, visceral, and neuropathic pain. The pain may also arise from incision, rib removal or damage, injury to the intercoastal nerve, pulmonary parenchyma incision and the presence or continuous irritation from chest tubes.

3. Postoperative pain after breast surgery

At some point in breast cancer treatment trajectory, patients may undergo surgery [15]. Hence, surgery is a treatment that has become the first line of approach against breast cancer. Surgery can be either breast conserving, such as lumpectomy, or a complete removal of all breast tissue, called mastectomy. The specific surgery depends on the stage and type of tumour a patient has [16]. Women with stage I, II, and III breast cancer can be treated with breast surgery including breast conserving surgery for stage I breast cancer and mastectomy for stage II and III breast cancer [17].

Irrespective of the type of breast surgery, patients experience postoperative pain. The pain responses usually stem from the surgical procedure itself. In the immediate postoperative period, the pain experienced by breast surgery patients is usually nociceptive and acute in nature and may be moderate or severe in nature [18]. Nociceptive pain is a type of pain that is characterised by localisation around the damaged tissue and resolves within the normal healing time [19], while acute pain is a type of pain characterised by sudden onset after tissue damage and high severity [18].

The nature of postoperative pain that occurs immediately after mastectomy is complex and multimodal in nature. For pain to be experienced, an external stimulus is usually transported via thin myelinated (i.e. A-δ fibres) and non-myelinated (i.e. C-fibres) fibres whose receptivity are determined by the control of sodium/calcium or potassium channels [20]. When the stimuli transported through C-fibres are more than those transported in A-δ fibres, little or no pain is experienced and vice versa [21]. This type of pain is constantly moderated by the brain stem and cortical pathways, and there may be a facilitation or inhibition of pain that further regulates both the sensory and emotional aspects of pain [19].

With pain after mastectomy, the severity experienced by individuals varies based on the degree of modification of the contact between the synapses, nociceptors, neurons at the dorsal horn of the spinal cord, and other nociceptive signal modulation structures in the central nervous system [20]. Depending on the severity of the pain, pain management regimen is prescribed [19] that may require the use of strong pain management regimen including opioids [22].

4. Impacts of postoperative pain on patients after thoracic and breast surgery

Postsurgical pain after surgery, sub-optimal or untreated pain has profound impacts or negative effects on patients. Pain after surgery usually and directly impedes respiratory function, mobilisation, delays recovery, increase duration of hospitalisation and hospital care costs of patient [6, 23–26].

The severity of pain is usually increased due to tension on the incision as a result of movement or mobilisation, deep breathing, and/or coughing [10, 11]. As a result, postoperative altered or impaired pulmonary function as well as postoperative pulmonary complications in postoperative patients is common and becomes the main clinical impact especially after thoracic surgery due to pre-existing lung disease, surgery-related loss of parenchyma, and inadequate postsurgical pain management [9, 27].

The surgical wound continuously moves as patients breathe, move, and cough, which worsens pain. Directly, pain impedes patient's performance of deep breathing which consequently limits inspiration, decreases lung compliance, and decreases functional residual capacity, thereby leading to postoperative atelectasis and hypoxemia [8, 10]. Likewise, ineffective coughing results in retention of secretions resulting in developing postoperative pneumonia [9, 11]. Furthermore, the development of shoulder pain causes patients to splint shoulder and decrease shoulder movement which impairs and causes gradual loss of both active and passive shoulder function [13, 28].

For most women who had undergone breast surgery, the impact of acute pain varies and may be dependent on whether the surgery is breast conserving or mastectomy with or without reconstruction. Additionally, psychosocial, physiological, and other individual risk factors contribute to the impact of pain on breast surgery patients [29]. A long-term impact of acute pain after breast surgery is the occurrence of persistent pain, which could result in negative health status and poor quality of life. If acute pain after breast surgery is inadequately managed, it may negatively impact sleep, work, interpersonal relationships, and activities of daily living [30].

5. Factors influencing acute pain after thoracic and breast surgery

Pain after breast and thoracic surgery is usually influenced by several factors that can be mainly categorised into patient factors, surgical approach, and analgesics technique factors [8, 14]. Previous studies have been conducted to examine determinants of pain after thoracic surgery. These are, however, mainly focused on determinants of post-thoracotomy pain syndrome or long-lasting pain after thoracic surgery [31].

5.1 Patient factors

A few studies have been done to determine how patient factors influence postsurgical pain intensity and response. Reports from the previous literature regarding gender differences and pain perception revealed female patients are less tolerant of noxious stimuli, frequently complain of severe and diffuse pain, and have higher risk for developing chronic pain than male patients [32, 33].

Age has also been identified in existing literature as a significant predictor of post-operative pain. The pharmacokinetics of pain medications can be affected by advanced age as the older adults are more sensitive to systemic opioids. For instance, a previous study revealed that elderly patients required 40% less amount of thoracic epidural analgesia because of the difference in thoracic epidural spread in the elderly [34]. A study conducted on 1231 patients to identify the risk factors contributing to postoperative pain in a referral hospital in developing country revealed younger age, female gender, and emergency surgery [35].

Another study conducted in a university hospital in Northeast Ethiopia showed American Society of Anaesthesiologists' Physical Status Classification System class I and II, general anaesthesia, and incision length exceeding 10 cm as risk factors contributing to postoperative pain [36]. Although younger age, being female, a history of depression and anxiety, and the lack of preoperative education about pain management are more likely to increase risks of severe acute post-surgical pain, a recent literature suggests that these risks have not been evidenced in thoracic surgery patients [37]. Furthermore, increased body mass index (BMI) has been recorded in a previous study to influence severity of pain as well as delay recovery after surgery [38]. To date, current evidence has been focused on predictors of persistent pain after thoracic and breast surgery with less attention to acute pain.

Since pain experience is subjective, sensory, and emotional, psychological factors can influence pain perception and pain experience. Pre-operative anxiety, depressive mood, and catastrophising have been shown to lower pain thresholds, thus predicting a more severe post-operative pain [14]. For this reason, assessment and management of patients' preoperative anxiety, depressive mood, catastrophising, and others negative moods become another essential role for nurses in preoperative preparedness. These require establishing good rapport and relationships with patient and family member, including implication of cognitive behavioural strategies and distraction techniques [14, 37].

Previous pain experience may influence the ways of thinking and responding or coping with pain after surgery. Patients who are vigilant or too concerned about pain and have negative thought or expectation about pain may influence the way they respond to pain or report worst pain after surgery. Furthermore, the past pain experience together with socio-cultural factors influences people on constructing certain assumptions, beliefs or myths, and attitudes about pain and pain medication [39]. In addition, experiences of pain medication used as well as existing pain before the present surgery and the previous surgeries have been recorded in literature as factors influencing pain after surgery. Use of opioids, anti-depressant, anti-convulsant, and the existing pain preoperatively, especially at a previous surgical site, are revealed as the predictors of moderate to severe postoperative pain [5].

The way people express pain or give meaning to their pain experience is partly influenced by their cultural background. Cultural stereotype conformed or shared by members of the same group passed from generation to generation affects pain expression in diverse ways. Often a patients' response to pain reflects whether they are members of a stoic or emotive culture. Stoic patients, mostly from African and Asian cultures, scarcely express their pain but "grin or bear it". In particular, the stoic culture promotes not drawing attention to ones' self, especially in a negative light [40]. Additionally, openly complaining or being assertive are considered inappropriate in a stoic culture while behaving in a dignified manner is considered appropriate. For this reason, although an individual feels pain, it is not culturally appropriate to express it [40]. Moreover, African and Asian patients will avoid making demands or questioning or bothering healthcare providers with complaints about pain. Meanwhile, emotive patients, mostly from Western cultures, are likely to verbalise their pain, prefer to have support around with an expectation that people react to their pain by validating what they are feeling [40].

Lastly, in some religion, pain acceptance hinged on a person's religious faith. For instance, Muslim patients may accept or reject pain medication based on their belief, and they could also consider their pain as God's blessing or believe that God can give them the ability to bear the pain. Meanwhile, Buddhists patients show stoicism when they experience pain and pain is viewed as common and accepting suffering leads to spiritual growth [40].

5.2 Surgical factors

The intensity of postoperative pain that a patient experience can be in part due to the technique used for the surgery [11]. Oftentimes, surgical methods or approaches that require more incisions or dissection of chest wall muscles can increase the postoperative pain intensity [11, 36]. Thoracic surgeries have been performed using several surgical techniques, and approaches mainly open thoracotomy and video-assisted thoracic surgery (VATS) [27, 41]. Although with open thoracotomy, reducing the size of the incision, using an appropriate muscle closing technique, or avoiding incising the latissimus dorsi may help reduce surgical tissue injury [11], VATS was created to limit the size of surgical incision and to avoid intercostal nerve damage in order to reduce pain after surgery [8, 11]. Thus, a longer incision and extended tissue trauma in open thoracotomy is expected to cause higher pain intensity compared with VATS [10]. Nevertheless, in women undergoing breast surgery, surgical techniques that require axillary lymph node dissection are predictive factors for severe postoperative pain [42].

6. Pharmacological pain management after thoracic and breast surgery

Current postoperative pain management methods have recommended the use of multimodal analgesia approaches to improve analgesic efficacy and minimise side effects. The multimodal analgesia is acknowledged in its significant role in all enhanced recovery after surgery pathways (ERAS) to manage pain, reduce stress responses, facilitate early mobilisation, and normal respiration [25, 43]. According to Montgomery and McNamara [44], multimodal analgesia has been acknowledged as effective pain management especially for preventing and controlling postsurgical pain as well as reducing side effects of opioid, hastening recovery, and shortening hospital stay. In the multimodal analgesia regimen, two or more analgesia and/or analgesic techniques with different mode or site of action are combined to produce more-effective analgesia than a unimodal regimen [25]. In multimodal approach, individual analgesia is recommended to be used at lower doses as this helps to reduce the side effects of each medication. Importantly, the central aim of multimodal analgesia is to avoid using opioids or reduce opioids consumption and thereby reduce the risk for opioids side effects that cause delay in recovery [25, 43].

For patients undergoing thoracic surgery, multimodal analgesia includes regional anaesthetic blockade in combination with using systemic nonopioid analgesia with opioid sparing [45]. Post-thoracic surgical pain therefore is expected to be treated with combinations of local anaesthetics, acetaminophen, non-steroidal anti-inflammatory drugs (NSAIDs), anticonvulsants, adrenergic agonists, and opioid-sparing methods [45–47].

Meanwhile for women undergoing breast surgery, typical pain management is a combination of opioids, non-opioids, non-pharmacological techniques, anaesthesia techniques, and patient-controlled analgesia techniques [47]. With these approaches, pain management can span through the intraoperative and postoperative periods. Intraoperatively, preventive pain medications employed for mastectomy patients include drugs such as nefopam, ketamine, and bupivacaine, with or without clonidine. All these medications have been reported to significantly reduce pain intensity after BC surgery, and they have long-term effects on pain experienced after surgery [48–51]. Moreover, the techniques employed in delivering the preventive medication (e.g. thoracic paravertebral block) reduced the pain score in one study [52], while a combination of paravertebral block with propofol significantly reduced the pain score in another study [53].

For both thoracic and breast surgery patients, the non-opioid drugs such as acetaminophen, NSAIDs, local anaesthetics, and anticonvulsants are combined with opioids-sparing analgesics or lower doses of opioids to manage postoperative pain [14, 25, 45]. These non-opioids limit the adverse effects of opioids including sedation, urine retention, nausea, pruritus vomiting, and slow gastrointestinal functioning in the multimodal regimen [46]. There is limited evidence about the recommended analgesic regimen for patients undergoing breast surgery in the ERAS pathway. However, the analgesics regimen recommended as multimodal analgesia for pain management in ERAS after thoracic surgery by Mehran et al. [45] are illustrated in **Figure 1**.

7. Non-pharmacological pain management after thoracic and breast surgery

Nonpharmacological interventions are essential to multimodal postoperative pain management and have been reported in the previous literatures to effectively relieve postoperative pain [54]. Notably, non-pharmacological pain management is not clearly presented in the existing pain management in an enhanced recovery pathways because it lacks high-quality evidence to support its use [44, 45]. According to clinical practice guidelines, non-pharmacological interventions are considered as adjunctive therapies of pharmacological interventions for postoperative pain management. These are transcutaneous electrical nerve stimulation (TENS), music therapy, cognitive–behavioural techniques, breathing relaxation technique, and cold therapy, massage, and acupuncture [47]. In accordance with the recommendations from national Centre for Complementary and Alternative Medicine about non-pharmacological pain management therapies for adults, the mechanism of each intervention is summarised in **Table 1**.

Non-pharmacological therapies can be beneficial in decreasing patients' pain [56], and they are suitable for use because they are non-invasive, have more benefits than harm and can be readily used by nurses [57]. However, consideration of patients' preference when using non-pharmacological interventions is essential [47, 58].

7.1 Preoperative education

Preoperative education is defined as the provision of information to patients awaiting surgery as a means of psychological preparation for surgery and the

- ➢ Gabapentin 300 mg orally three times a day for 30 days
- ➢ Use the pediatric dosage (100 mg three times a day) for geriatric patients or those experiencing lightheadedness
- ➢ Acetaminophen 1,000 mg IV every 6 hours for 48 hours, then 1,000 mg orally every 6 hours
- ➢ Ketorolac 15 mg IV every 6 hours for 48 hours (if not contraindicated)
- ➢ Celecoxib 200 mg orally twice a day
- ➢ Famotidine 40 mg orally twice a day while receiving Ketorolac or Celebrex
- ➢ Tramadol 50 mg orally every 6 hours as needed as first rescue medication if the patient reports a pain score higher than 4 on a 10-point scale
- ➢ Hydromorphone 0.5 mg IV every 15 minutes up to 2 times as needed as second rescue medication if the pain is not relieved with tramadol
- ➢ If pain persists, a patient-controlled anesthesia pump with hydromorphone
- ➢ Ondansetron 4 mg IV every 6 hours as needed for nausea
- ➢ Controlled with celecoxib, acetaminophen, and gabapentin and continued at discharge, along with tramadol 50 mg orally 4 times a day as needed
- ➢ For breakthrough pain, patients who require rescue hydromorphone are discharged with the above medications and a prescription for a hydromorphone 2 mg orally every 4 hours as needed
- ➢ A dedicated follow-up nurse calls for all patients within 72 hours to address issues associated with pain and wound care

Figure 1.
Pain management in an enhanced recovery pathway after thoracic surgery according to Mehran et al. [45].

Non-pharmacological method	Mechanism
Preoperative education	
Acupuncture	Balances energy channels in the body that helps reduce pain
Relaxation therapies (music, meditation, aromatherapy)	Help increase energy levels and improve mood that trigger body to release endorphins
Physical therapies (massage, cold and ice application)	Relax tight muscles and decrease pain, swelling and may prevent tissue damage
Transcutaneous electrical nerve stimulation	Reduce muscle spasm and soft tissue oedema

Table 1.
Mechanism of action for various non-pharmacological methods. Adapted from national centre for complementary and integrative health (NCCIH) [55].

postsurgical recovery process [59]. Preoperative education is one of the most effective ways to control anxiety in patients awaiting surgery [60], and it serves to enhance patient involvement in their postoperative pain management through informed decision-making [47, 61]. Additionally, preoperative education allows the patient to adequately prepare for the surgery and to manage postoperative pain effectively [60].

The information provided during preoperative education usually covers the surgical process, anaesthesia, pain, and what to expect after surgery [62–64].

The key thing to remember is preoperative preparedness as well as preoperative education and counselling for appropriate pain relief and control after surgery [8, 47]. Before surgery, according to Chou and colleagues, individualised and family-oriented education as well as mutual goal setting should be allocated in relation to appropriate pain relief after surgery [47]. For instance, education about types of pain, sources of pain, when and how to report pain using pain chart, pain medications commonly used, and side effects should be included in preoperative teaching [47].

Adequate information regarding pain assessment, proposed analgesic medication and technique, complications, and its management are recommended whenever possible [8]. The patient education does not exclude non-pharmacological pain management methods or techniques according to preference of each individual patient (e.g. massage, music therapy, cold application, and distraction techniques). Encouragements to use and choose a preferred non-pharmacological therapy in combination with skill development are also performed preoperatively [46, 47]. Oftentimes, surgery-related information is provided by surgeons. However, it is more effective when the anaesthesiologist also provides patients with information related to anaesthesia alongside the information provided by the surgeon [65]. According to Chou and colleagues, effective preoperative education should include detailed information related to treatment options, type of pain, expectations, and goal setting for the pain intensity the client intend to achieve postoperatively [47]. The information that is included in a preoperative education is especially important for younger women because they have higher risk for severe postoperative pain [37].

The effectiveness of preoperative teaching using a variety of teaching strategies has been examined by the previous studies, which revealed the benefit of it [59, 66, 67]. According to Ramesh and colleagues, patients who are well informed before surgery tend to experience little pain [59]. Preoperative education can be delivered to patients individually or in groups [60] through face-to-face sessions or technological devices [47]. Information can be provided by lecture, booklets, pamphlets, videos, audiotapes, and technology-assisted devices [47, 68]. Written information can also be used to reinforce information provided verbally to patients and vice versa [60, 64]. Using either of these means, preoperative education can be provided to different surgical patients.

Irrespective of the patient education method chosen, delivering the information too quickly and inadequately can hinder the patient's understanding of and the sufficiency of the information, as well as their satisfaction with the preoperative education [60]. This includes patients awaiting all types of surgery [66], knee surgery [64], spinal surgery [62], cardiac surgery [61, 69, 70], abdominal surgery [71], renal surgery [63] and breast cancer surgery [72]. Most of the studies reported that preoperative education was effective in controlling anxiety in patients awaiting surgery and pain after surgery.

7.2 Acupuncture

Acupuncture is a non-pharmacological intervention that helps to reduce pain by stimulating specific nerve points called acupoints. Acupoints are a few dynamic, complex structures that consist of blood vessels, mast cells, and nerve fibres [73]. The acupoints are reached with the help of thin, solid metallic needles that penetrate the skin. Acupuncture technique has been used in Asia for thousands of years as part of traditional Chinese, Japanese, and Korean medicine [74]. Acupuncture can be delivered as manual acupuncture or electroacupuncture [73, 74]. Manual acupuncture is conducted by inserting the needle into the skin at the corresponding acupoint, and then, the needle is moved in different direction to stimulate the acupoint mechanically. Meanwhile for electroacupuncture, mechanical and electrical stimulations of acupoints are achieved by passing electric currents through acupuncture needles [73].

Acupuncture is believed to be governed by three main principles which are modulating yin and yang, differentiating between primary and secondary *Qi* (i.e. vital energy), and inhibiting pathogenicity and enhancing immunity [75]. The achievement of these main principles is based on the theory of meridians, collaterals, and acupoints. Meridians ("Jing and Luo", 'links or connection') are the transport pathways for *Qi* and blood, controlling yin and yang, connecting Zang organs with Fu organs, and connecting the external and internal as well as the upper and lower body of humans [76]. Collaterals are thin networks of small interwoven channels that run throughout the body [75]. According to this theory, diseases are treatable through acupoints as they are closest to the body's surface. Through acupoints, meridian obstructions can be removed, *Qi* and blood can be controlled, inadequacies can be reinforced, and excesses can be curtailed [76].

Although acupuncture's mode of action in pain relief is not fully understood, some studies have posited that acupuncture triggers the release of endogenous opioids and neurotransmitters that are responsible for pain control [77]. Pain control begins at the acupoint where acupuncture-induced signals are generated and transmitted to the brain via the spinal cord. As the signals reach the brain, there is a rise or decline in many neurotransmitters, inflammatory factors, and pain relief modulators [73]. The ability of acupuncture to control pain depends on acupuncture manipulation, sensation, acupoint, pathological status, and the type of pain [78].

In general, the effectiveness of acupuncture has been widely contested because its mechanism is yet to be fully understood [79]. However, some systematic reviews have reported that acupuncture is effective in relieving cancer pain [80, 81], low back pain [82–84] and postoperative pain [85–87]. For women who have undergone mastectomy, acupuncture was used in one study for acute pain management and was found to be effective [77].

8. Relaxation therapies

Relaxation therapies have also been recommended for pain management after surgery [46, 47]. A few interventions belong to this group of therapies because they share some similar components and requires patient's acceptance and rapport building before its initiation [46]. These interventions include breathing exercises, music therapy, aromatherapy, and meditation [5, 46, 47].

Previous studies about relaxation therapies have focused on music therapy [88, 89], meditation [90, 91], and aromatherapy [92, 93]. These studies have supported that after breast or thoracic surgery, relaxation therapies reduce pain intensity as well as pain distress at rest, during deep breathing and turning.

8.1 Music interventions

The history of utilising music for healthcare purposes dates to the sixth century. However, Florence Nightingale recognised its importance in the clinical area in the eighteenth century [94]. Since then, music has been widely used for anxiety reduction and pain management across various patient populations—including preoperative and postoperative patients—because it is not physically or cognitively tasking [95]. Music has also been used to control blood pressure, respiratory rates, and heart rates of various groups of patients because it promotes relaxation [5, 96–99].

The way patients respond to music differs and is mainly dependent on the patients' knowledge about the music, culture, environment, and preferences [100]. Finlay and Anil concluded in their study that the types of music that have been successfully used to improve patient outcomes include music that the listener is familiar with, prefers, and can resonate with emotionally [101], because personal preferences and familiarity can stimulate attention to the music, thus distracting patients [102].

The positive effects of music on anxiety are made possible through distraction, which occurs when lyrics or the sound of familiar music occupies the attention centre of the brain, creating meaningful auditory stimuli [100]. However, the precise mechanism of pain reduction that music elicits is not widely understood [103], though the benefits have been established through research [104]. One of the methods that music is believed to use to relieve pain is inherent in the cognitive and emotional characteristics it possesses, which allows it to act as an external and distracting stimulus [102].

Music can be used passively through listening to downloaded songs or songs on compact discs or actively through singing and drumming [100, 105]. Beyond the familiarity, culture, and environment of the patients and the mode of music delivery (i.e. active or passive), music has six main components that also influence patient's response to music. Each of these components is processed by the brain through different pathways [106]. These components include volume, tempo, rhythm, pitch, melody, and timbre. Controlling these components will result in either relaxing music or stimulating music [107], which will have different effects on patients, depending on their preference and familiarity with the music [108]. To further enhance the effectiveness of music in clinical settings, music should be set at 60 to 80 beats per minute [109], and patients should be allowed to control the volume of the music [105]. Music should also be played for 20 to 60 minutes on portable devices for individuals or public address systems for groups [100, 105, 109].

Evidence from the previous literature has revealed that music is beneficial to patients experiencing pain [106, 110], and music is effective in reducing pain among cancer patients [111] and patients awaiting surgery [112]. Previous studies have also reported that music is effective in reducing pain in patients who have undergone a bone marrow transplant [113] and knee surgery [114]. For patients undergoing breast cancer surgery, a recent systematic review also reported that music interventions effectively reduced acute postoperative pain [87].

8.2 Meditation

Meditation is the process of training one's attention and consciousness via the voluntary regulation of mental processes [115]. Meditation is an important method of understanding the nature of the mind and a means to attain a certain degree of consciousness. Meditation is a common religious practice in both the East and West. The techniques used in the East and West are similar, including "breath-oriented multitasking meditation", mindfulness meditation, and relaxation response [116]. Meditation involves a self-regulatory process that can improve symptoms through the maintenance of the balance of autonomic responses [117]. These responses include improved vital signs (i.e. pulse rate and blood pressure), cardiac activities, and oxygen consumption [116], all of which are cardinal consequences of inadequate anxiety and pain management.

Meditation as a non-pharmacological intervention engages three main structures in the brain, including the anterior cingulate cortex, the anterior insula, and the ventromedial prefrontal cortices [118, 119]. A steady practice of meditation results in higher activities at the ventromedial prefrontal cortices, causing a greater level of anxiety reduction [119]. Meanwhile, when meditation is used for pain management, the three main structures interact with pain in the limbic–thalamic region because both pain and meditation elicit affective, sensory, and cognitive responses [118]. This interaction results in the activation of the endogenous opioid system [120].

Although meditation has three main techniques, the most commonly researched one is mindfulness meditation. In general, meditation has been found to be effective in reducing anxiety in patients undergoing cardiac surgery [121] and for pain management in patients with cancer, fibromyalgia, migraines, and irritable bowel syndrome [122], as well as for patients after abdominal surgery [91]. However, there is limited evidence on its use after breast surgery, thus creating a dearth in evidence on its effectiveness for postoperative pain management in patients undergoing breast surgery.

8.3 Aromatherapy

Aromatherapy is a botanical therapy that reinforces the therapeutic value of smell and sometimes touch during care delivery [123]. The botanical nature of this therapy involves the use of plant oil for health purposes. According to Tamaki and colleagues, aromatherapy is the application of extracted essential oils—from flowers, herbs, and other parts of the plant—to treat different illnesses [124]. The use of aromatherapy has a long history as it was practiced in ancient Mesopotamia, Egypt, China, Greece, Rome, and Israel. However, modern-day aromatherapy was developed by a French scientist who accidentally dipped his burnt hand into a jar of lavender oil, and the wound healed rapidly without a scar. Since then, modern medicine has researched the use of essential oils for health purposes [125].

Although aromatherapy's mechanism of action has been widely contested by different scientists, most believe that the link between the olfactory and limbic systems is the main pathway for its action of influencing mood and emotions [126]. Once the odour of an essential oil binds to a certain protein in the olfactory cells, it stimulates the olfactory nerve, which transmits a signal to the limbic system and the hypothalamus [125]. In the limbic system, the amygdala, which controls emotional responses, and the hippocampus, which controls explicit memory formation and retrieval, then transmit a signal to the cerebral cortex. The cerebral cortex allows interaction between thoughts and feelings and the brain centre that controls stress and hormone levels and vital signs [123]. Aside from the assimilation of essential oil through the olfactory system, it can also be assimilated through the skin and mucous membranes by diffusion [123, 125, 127, 128]. However, inhalation appears to provide the most rapid effect. Similarly, it is believed that the chemical properties and composition of an essential oil are what determines how effective a specific type of oil may be [123]. According to Halcon, there are various essential oils that can be used when delivering aromatherapy, but the commonest essential oil used in the previous studies was lavender oil through inhalation [123].

In the clinical setting, aromatherapy has been mainly used to manage pain, anxiety, agitation, nausea, and insomnia and to prevent infection. For each symptom, the mode of application may vary from inhalation and ingestion to topical application [123]. However, most of the previous research has focused on the use of aromatherapy to control stress symptoms, especially anxiety among various patient populations including patients waiting for surgery [129–131]. This can be due to the already established understanding of the connection between aromatherapy and the limbic system, which is the centre of emotions. Meanwhile, some other studies have been conducted to test the effects of aromatherapy on the mood and pain of patients undergoing various breast cancer treatments including surgery and thoracic surgery [124, 132–137].

8.4 Physical therapies

8.4.1 Massage

Massage belongs to the group of physical therapies, and it is seen as essential to health and well-being [138] which provides pain relief either during or immediately after the intervention [47]. Massage is the use of manual methods and adjunctive treatments to positively affect patient's health and well-being. The root word of massage is from the Arabic word "mass'h", which means "press gently" [139]. Massage has gained widespread popularity for preoperative anxiety management [140] and for pain management among hospitalised patients [90, 141]. However, massage has been mostly used for pain management [142]. Massage provides relief for anxiety and pain, but its mechanism of action is yet to be understood [143]. Many scientists have suggested that massage works to relieve anxiety by promoting relaxation [139] and working on the subconscious mind to promote positive emotions [144]. Likewise, massage can relieve pain by producing a localised effect on muscles [144] and by activating non-myelinated C-fibres which inhibits the perception of pain [139].

Massage can be provided in the hospital, and it has yielded a considerable level of positive effects [145]. There are various types of massage techniques that have evolved from different cultures. The taxonomy of these techniques is based on both Western massage and Eastern massage. Eastern massage technique includes Thai massage, reflexology, acupressure, shiatsu, polarity therapy, and others. Meanwhile, Western massage technique includes Swedish, myofascial, reflexive, soft-tissue release, circulatory, lymphatic, neuromuscular massage, and others [144]. Different massage techniques may produce different effects or expected outcomes in patients. However, for pain management, patient involvement in the decision-making process about where to massage, as well as patient assessment prior to massage, may help to increase the positive effects of massage [145]. Despite the popularity of massage for pain management among postoperative patients who have undergone cardiac surgery [140, 145–149] and thoracic surgery [141, 150], only a few types of massage have been used for pain management in women undergoing breast surgery. The studies conducted among thoracic and breast surgery patients found that massage can be used routinely in the hospital to help patients who have undergone mastectomy or breast cancer surgery control their pain better [90, 140–142, 146, 151, 152].

8.4.2 Cold applications

Application of cold on the skin which may need a compression or an equipment that can recirculate mechanically for cold temperature maintenance is described as cold therapy [47]. Cold therapy is a common nursing intervention and has proven effective in most surgeries especially open-heart surgeries by reducing patient's incisional pain [153].

Application of cold therapy is common in acute pain settings including postoperative pain settings, and its effect has been identified to be related to tissue temperature reduction at the surgical which results in localised pain relief and oedema reduction [153]. Previous studies have recorded success in the use of cold therapy in pain management after thoracic surgery. Ice pack placed on incision site reduced pain in the previous studies by reducing the temperature at the surgical site, numbness, and promoting feeling of coolness [153–156]. The implementation of cold therapy by nurses can be done independently, and patient's acceptability is feasible because it is cost-effective and easy to use [154].

8.5 Transcutaneous electrical nerve stimulation

Transcutaneous electrical nerve stimulation (TENS) is a non-pharmacological intervention that utilises low electrical currents on intact skin to stimulate nerve activities that inhibit or enhance certain nerve impulses [157]. TENS was basically developed for pain relief; however, it also enhances venous haemostasis through motor and skeletal nerve stimulation [158, 159]. TENS is an intervention that has been delivered by many healthcare providers, including nurses, because it is safe, cheap, non-invasive, and does not require physician expertise [157]. The mechanism of action of TENS is based on the gate control theory developed by Melzack [160]. TENS activates the descending inhibitory pain pathway [158] by first activating the large unmyelinated A-β fibres that prevent noxious stimuli transmission [161]. When TENS is delivered at a high frequency, certain receptors in the bloodstream (i.e. beta-endorphins) and cerebrospinal fluid (i.e. methionine-enkephalin) increase in concentration creating a myriad of opioid-receptor blockades in the rostral ventromedial medulla and the spinal cord [161].

According to Vance and colleagues, TENS has been utilised for pain management in various patient populations including patients with neck cancer, those with phantom limb pain, those undergoing labour, and those who have undergone thoracic surgery [161]. TENS has also been tested in patients undergoing cardiac surgery. Nonetheless, there are inconsistent findings on the effects of TENS on pain after surgery [158]. There is also a lack of evidence on the utilisation of TENS for anxiety prevention and in women undergoing breast cancer surgery. However, TENS may be beneficial in reducing pain in patients with undergoing breast surgery.

9. Conclusion

This chapter has elaborated the mechanisms of postoperative pain after thoracic and breast surgery, which is generally short-term and acute in nature. Inadequate pain management can exert profound and negative impacts on the recovery of patients. In addition, various patient factors and surgical factors not only predict the development and intensity of postsurgical pain, but also influence how patient responds or copes with pain after surgery. To promote the recovery after surgery, both pharmacological and non-pharmacological pain relief methods are recommended to be integrated as a multimodal pain management plan for patient awaiting surgery. Indeed, adequate, and effective multimodal pain management plans require appropriate regimen and dose of individual analgesic agents to minimise the side effects of medication, as well as tailored non-pharmacological therapies that consider patient's preference. For future research, high-quality experimental studies are warranted to provide evidence on the delivery of non-pharmacological therapies among different populations within their unique social and cultural contexts. Moreover, exploring the mechanisms of non-pharmacological therapies on pain relief is needed to enhance the potential effects of such therapies. To enhance pain management in clinical praxis, the selection and delivery of pain management therapies should consider patient factors, especially patients' preference, to promote the efficacy of their multimodal pain management plans.

Acknowledgements

YOT would like to acknowledge the support of Assistant Professor Khomapak Maneewat for contributing to the development of the idea for the non-pharmacological management of thoracic surgery.

Conflict of interest

The authors declare no conflict of interest.

Author details

Yetunde Oluwafunmilayo Tola[1,2,3*], Ka Ming Chow[1*], Wei Liang[1,4], Esther Ilesanmi[3,5], Oluwatosin Comfort Olarinde[3,5] and Deborah Blessing Odejobi[3,5]

1 The Nethersole School of Nursing, Faculty of Medicine, Chinese University of Hong Kong, Hong Kong (SAR), China

2 Faculty of Nursing, Prince of Songkla University, Hat Yai, Thailand

3 Institute of Nursing Research, Osogbo, Osun State, Nigeria

4 School of Nursing, Nanjing Medical University, Nanjing, China

5 Faculty of Nursing, Ladoke Akintola University of Technology, Ogbomoso, Nigeria

*Address all correspondence to: tolayetunde702@link.cuhk.edu.hk
and kmchow@cuhk.edu.hk

References

[1] Wooden SR. Chronic postsurgical pain. Annual Review of Nursing Research. 2016;**35**:91–X

[2] Sobol-Kwapinska M, Bąbel P, Plotek W, et al. Psychological correlates of acute postsurgical pain: A systematic review and meta-analysis. European Journal of Pain (United Kingdom). 2016;**20**:1573-1586

[3] Humble SR, Dalton AJ, Li L. A systematic review of therapeutic interventions to reduce acute and chronic post-surgical pain after amputation, thoracotomy or mastectomy. European Journal of Pain. 2015;**19**:451-465

[4] Odejobi YO, Maneewat K, Chittithavorn V. Nurse-led post-thoracic surgery pain management programme: Its outcomes in a Nigerian hospital. International Nursing Review. 2019;**66**:434-441

[5] Liu Y, Petrini MA. Effects of music therapy on pain, anxiety, and vital signs in patients after thoracic surgery. Complementary Therapies in Medicine. 2015;**23**:714-718

[6] Darr C, Cheufou D, Weinreich G, et al. Robotic thoracic surgery results in shorter hospital stay and lower postoperative pain compared to open thoracotomy: A matched pairs analysis. Surgical Endoscopy. 2017;**31**:4126-4130. DOI: 10.1007/s00464-017-5464-6

[7] Kol E, Erdogan A, Karslı B. Nature and intensity of the pain following thoracotomy. International Journal of Nursing Practice. 2012;**18**:84-90

[8] Mesbah A, Yeung J, Gao F. Pain after thoracotomy. BJA Education. 2016;**16**:1-7

[9] Attri JP, Kaur R, Kaur H, et al. Post thoracotomy pain management: A review of current available modalities. Northern Journal of ISA. 2016;**1**:7-10

[10] Kolettas A, Lazaridis G, Baka S, et al. Postoperative pain management. Journal of Thoracic Disease. 2015;**7**:S62-S72

[11] Sungur MO, Şentürk M. Pain management following thoracic surgery. In: Şentürk M, Orhan Sungur M, editors. Postoperative Care in Thoracic Surgery: A Comprehensive Guide. Cham: Springer International Publishing. pp. 243-257

[12] Brennan TJ. Pathophysiology of postoperative pain. Pain. 2011;**152**:S33-S40

[13] Blichfeldt-Eckhardt MR, Laursen CB, Berg H, et al. A randomised, controlled, double-blind trial of ultrasound-guided phrenic nerve block to prevent shoulder pain after thoracic surgery. Anaesthesia. 2016;**71**:1441-1448

[14] Tan M, Law LS, Gan TJ. Optimizing pain management to facilitate enhanced recovery after surgery pathways. Canadian Journal of Anesthesia; Toronto. 2015;**62**:203-218

[15] Schreiber JA, Cantrell D, Moe KA, et al. Improving knowledge, assessment, and attitudes related to pain management: Evaluation of an intervention. Pain Management Nursing. 2014;**15**:474-481

[16] Fraser VJ, Nickel KB, Fox IK, et al. The epidemiology and outcomes of breast cancer surgery. Transactions of the American Clinical and Climatological Association. 2016;**127**:46-58

[17] American Cancer Society. Treatment of breast cancer stages I–III. 2019. Available from: https://www.cancer.org/cancer/breast-cancer/treatment/

treatment-of-breast-cancer-by-stage/treatment-of-breast-cancer-stages-i-iii.html [Accessed: August 12, 2020]

[18] Abd-Elsayed A, Deer TR. Different types of pain. In: Abd-Elsayed A, editor. Pain. Cham: Springer; 2019. DOI: 10.1007/978-3-319-99124-5_3

[19] Chimenti RL, Frey-Law LA, Sluka KA. A mechanism-based approach to physical therapist management of pain. Physical Therapy. 2018;**98**:302-314

[20] Vardeh D, Mannion RJ, Woolf CJ. Toward a mechanism-based approach to pain diagnosis. The Journal of Pain. 2016;**17**:T50-T69

[21] McMahon SB, Koltzenburg M, Tracey I, et al. Wall & Melzack's Textbook of Pain. Philadelphia: Elsevier Health Sciences; 2013. Available from: https://books.google.co.th/books?id=ok0_jIJ0w_wC

[22] Baron RH. Surgical management of breast cancer. Seminars in Oncology Nursing. 2007;**23**:10-19

[23] Ardò NP, Loizzi D, Panariti S, et al. Enhanced recovery pathways in thoracic surgery from Italian VATS group: Nursing care program. Journal of Thoracic Disease. 2018;**10**:S529-S534

[24] Bendixen M, Jørgensen OD, Kronborg C, et al. Postoperative pain and quality of life after lobectomy via video-assisted thoracoscopic surgery or anterolateral thoracotomy for early-stage lung cancer: A randomised controlled trial. The Lancet Oncology. 2016;**17**:836-844

[25] Starkweather A, Perry M. Enhanced recovery programs and pain management. Topics in Pain Management. 2017;**32**:1-9

[26] Zvara DA. Enhanced recovery for thoracic surgery. Revista Mexicana de Anestesiología. 2017;**40**:340-344

[27] Lazopoulos A, Barbetakis N, Lazaridis G, et al. Open thoracotomy for pneumothorax. Journal of Thoracic Disease. 2015;**7**:S50-S55

[28] Wolin PM, Ingraffia-Welp A, Moreyra CE, et al. High-intensity stretch treatment for severe postoperative adhesive capsulitis of the shoulder. Annals of Physical and Rehabilitation Medicine. 2016;**59**:242-247

[29] Schreiber KL, Zinboonyahgoon N, Xu X, et al. Preoperative psychosocial and psychophysical phenotypes as predictors of acute pain outcomes after breast surgery. The Journal of Pain. 2019;**20**:540-556

[30] Villa G, Mandarano R, Scirè-Calabrisotto C, et al. Chronic pain after breast surgery: Incidence, associated factors, and impact on quality of life, an observational prospective study. Perioperative Medicine. 2021;**10**:1-11

[31] Macrea LM, Maurer K. Post-thoracotomy pain syndrome: PTPS. In: Yong RJ, Nguyen M, Nelson E, et al., editors. Pain Medicine: An Essential Review. Cham: Springer International Publishing. pp. 489-490

[32] Breivik H, Skovlund E. More postoperative pain reported by women than by men—Again. Scandinavian Journal of Pain. 2016;**12**:96-97

[33] Storesund A, Krukhaug Y, Olsen MV, et al. Females report higher postoperative pain scores than males after ankle surgery. Scandinavian Journal of Pain. 2016;**12**:85-93

[34] Zheng H, Schnabel A, Yahiaoui-Doktor M, Meissner W, van Aken H, Zahn P, et al. Age and preoperative pain are major confounders for sex differences in postoperative pain outcome: A prospective database analysis. PLoS One. 2017;**12**(6):1-14

[35] Murray AA, Retief FW. Acute postoperative pain in 1 231 patients at a developing country referral hospital: Incidence and risk factors. Southern African Journal of Anaesthesia and Analgesia. 2016;**22**:19-24

[36] Admassu WS, Hailekiros AG, Abdissa ZD. Severity and risk factors of post-operative pain in university of Gondar hospital, northeast Ethiopa. Journal of Anesthesia & Clinical Research. 2016;**7**. Epub ahead of print 2016. DOI: 10.4172/2155-6148.1000675

[37] Hegarty D. Post thoracotomy pain syndrome: What pain management options do we have? Journal of Surgery & Transplantation Science. 2017;**3**:1059

[38] Viscusi ER, Ding L, Phipps JB, et al. High body mass index and use of fentanyl iontophoretic transdermal system in postoperative pain management: Results of a pooled analysis of six phase 3/3B trials. Pain and therapy. 2016;**6**:29-43

[39] Linton SJ, Shaw WS. Impact of psychological factors in the experience of pain. Physical Therapy. 2011;**91**:700-711

[40] Narayan MC. Culture's effects on pain assessment and management. AJN, American Journal of Nursing. 2010;**110**:38-47

[41] Brunelli A, Falcoz PE, D'Amico T, et al. European guidelines on structure and qualification of general thoracic surgery. European Journal of Cardio-Thoracic Surgery. 2014;**45**:779-786

[42] Wang L, Guyatt GH, Kennedy SA, et al. Predictors of persistent pain after breast cancer surgery: A systematic review and meta-analysis of observational studies. CMAJ. 2016;**188**:E352-E361

[43] Beverly A, Kaye AD, Ljungqvist O, et al. Essential elements of multimodal analgesia in enhanced recovery after surgery (ERAS) guidelines. Anesthesiology Clinics. 2017;**35**:e115-e143

[44] Montgomery R, McNamara SA. Multimodal pain management for enhanced recovery: Reinforcing the shift from traditional pathways through nurse-led interventions. AORN Journal. 2016;**104**:S9-S16

[45] Mehran RJ, Martin LW, Baker CM, et al. Pain management in an enhanced recovery pathway after thoracic surgical procedures. The Annals of Thoracic Surgery. 2016;**102**:e595-e596

[46] Schug SA, Palmer GM, Scott DA, et al. Acute pain management: Scientific evidence, fourth edition. Medical Journal of Australia. 2015;**204**. Available from: https://www.mja.com.au/journal/2016/204/8/acute-pain-management-scientific-evidence-fourth-edition-2015

[47] Chou R, Gordon DB, de Leon-Casasola OA, et al. Management of postoperative pain: A clinical practice guideline from the American pain society, the American society of regional anesthesia and pain medicine, and the American society of anesthesiologists' committee on regional anesthesia, executive committee, and administrative council. Journal of Pain. 2016;**17**:131-157

[48] Cho A-R, Kwon J-Y, Kim K-H, et al. The effects of anesthetics on chronic pain after breast cancer surgery: Anesthesia and analgesia. Anesthesia & Analgesic. 2013;**116**:683-693

[49] Mcnicol ED, Schumann R, Haroutounian S. A systematic review and meta-analysis of ketamine for the prevention of persistent post-surgical pain. Acta Anaesthesiologica Scandinavica. 2014;**58**:1199-1213

[50] Mohamed SA-B, Abdel-Ghaffar HS. Effect of the addition of clonidine to locally administered bupivacaine on acute and chronic postmastectomy pain. Journal of Clinical Anesthesia; Philadelphia. 2013;**25**:20-27

[51] Na H-S, Oh A-Y, Koo B-W, et al. Preventive analgesic efficacy of nefopam in acute and chronic pain after breast cancer surgery. Medicine. 2016;**95**. Epub ahead of print 9 February 2016. DOI: 10.1097/MD.0000000000003705

[52] Agarwal RR, Wallace AM, Madison SJ, et al. Single-injection thoracic paravertebral block and postoperative analgesia after mastectomy: A retrospective cohort study. Journal of Clinical Anesthesia; Philadelphia. 2015;**27**:371-374

[53] Wu J, Buggy D, Fleischmann E, et al. Thoracic paravertebral regional anesthesia improves analgesia after breast cancer surgery: A randomized controlled multicentre clinical trial. Canadian Journal of Anesthesia; Toronto. 2015;**62**:241-251

[54] Manworren RCB. Multimodal pain management and the future of a personalized medicine approach to pain. AORN Journal. 2015;**101**:307-318

[55] NCCIH. Clinical Practice Guidelines. National Centre for Complemntary and Integrative Health. 2018. Available from: https://nccih.nih.gov/health/providers/clinicalpractice.htm

[56] Saadatmand V, Rejeh N, Heravi-Karimooi M, et al. Effects of natural sounds on pain: A randomized controlled trial with patients receiving mechanical ventilation support. Pain Management Nursing. 2015;**16**:483-492

[57] Salmani F, Abadi A, Taheri SM, et al. Effect of beloved person's voice on chest tube removal pain in patients undergoing open heart surgery: Fuzzy logistic regression model. Journal of Paramedical Sciences. 2017;**8**:46-51

[58] Czarnecki ML, Turner HN, Collins PM, et al. Procedural pain management: A position statement with clinical practice recommendations. Pain Management Nursing. 2011;**12**:95-111

[59] Ramesh C, Nayak BS, Pai VB, et al. Effect of preoperative education on postoperative outcomes among patients undergoing cardiac surgery: A systematic review and meta-analysis. Journal of Perianesthesia Nursing. 2017;**32**:518-529.e2

[60] Akyüz E, Erdem Y. Patients' experiences of informed consent and preoperative education. Clinical Nursing Research. 2021;**30**:529-538

[61] Hoseini S, Soltani F, Beygi MB, et al. The effect of educational audiotape programme on anxiety and depression in patients undergoing coronary artery bypass graft. Journal of Clinical Nursing. 2013;**22**:1613-1619

[62] Eastwood D, Manson N, Bigney E, et al. Improving postoperative patient reported benefits and satisfaction following spinal fusion with a single preoperative education session. The Spine Journal. 2019;**19**:840-845

[63] Teishima J, Takayama Y, Iwaguro S, et al. Usefulness of personalized three-dimensional printed model on the satisfaction of preoperative education for patients undergoing robot-assisted partial nephrectomy and their families. International Urology and Nephrology. 2018;**50**:1061-1066

[64] Kelmer GC, Turcotte JJ, Dolle SS, et al. Preoperative education for total joint arthroplasty: Does reimbursement reduction threaten improved

outcomes? The Journal of Arthroplasty. 2021;**36**:2651-2657

[65] Rachman S. Anxiety. 2nd ed. Hove: New York: Psychology Press; Taylor & Francis; 2004

[66] van Dijk JFM, van Wijck AJM, Kappen TH, et al. The effect of a preoperative educational film on patients' postoperative pain in relation to their request for opioids. Pain Management Nursing. 2015;**16**:137-145

[67] Watt-Watson J, Stevens B, Costello J, et al. Impact of preoperative education on pain management outcomes after coronary artery bypass graft surgery: A pilot. Canadian Journal of Nursing Research Archive. 2016;**31**:41-56. Available from: http://cjnr.archive.mcgill.ca/article/view/1550

[68] Kühlmann AYR, de Rooij A, Kroese LF, et al. Meta-analysis evaluating music interventions for anxiety and pain in surgery. British Journal of Surgery. 2018;**105**:773-783

[69] Géraldine CJ, Racine M, et al. Web-based nursing intervention for self-management of pain after cardiac surgery: Pilot randomized controlled trial. Journal of Medical Internet Research. 2012;**14**(6):e177 https://www.jmir.org/2012/6/e177

[70] Kalogianni A, Almpani P, Vastardis L, et al. Can nurse-led preoperative education reduce anxiety and postoperative complications of patients undergoing cardiac surgery? European Journal of Cardiovascular Nursing. 2016;**15**:447-458

[71] Best JT, Musgrave B, Pratt K, et al. The impact of scripted pain education on patient satisfaction in outpatient abdominal surgery patients. Journal of Perianesthesia Nursing. 2018;**33**:453-460

[72] Sayin Y, Aksoy G. The effect of analgesic education on pain in patients undergoing breast surgery: Within 24 hours after the operation. Journal of Clinical Nursing. 2012;**21**:1244-1253

[73] Chen T, Zhang WW, Chu YX, et al. Acupuncture for pain management: Molecular mechanisms of action. American Journal of Chinese Medicine. 2020;**48**:793-811

[74] Greenlee H, Balneaves LG, Carlson LE, et al. Clinical practice guidelines on the use of integrative therapies as supportive care in patients treated for breast cancer. Journal of the National Cancer Institute. Monographs. 2014;**2014**:346-358

[75] Cao X. History of modern acupuncture research in China. In: Acupuncture Therapy for Neurological Diseases: A Neurobiological View. 2010. pp. 1-31

[76] Zhou F, Huang D, YingXia. Neuroanatomic basis of acupuncture points. In: Xia Y, Cao X, Wu G, Cheng J, editors. Acupuncture Therapy for Neurological Diseases. Berlin, Heidelberg: Springer; 2010. DOI: 10.1007/978-3-642-10857-0_2

[77] Quinlan-Woodward J, Gode A, Dusek JA, et al. Assessing the impact of acupuncture on pain, nausea, anxiety, and coping in women undergoing a mastectomy. Oncology Nursing Forum. 2016;**43**:725-732

[78] Xiang A, Cheng K, Shen X, Xu P, Liu S. The immediate analgesic effect of acupuncture for pain: A systematic review and meta-analysis. Evidence-Based Complementary and Alternative Medicine. 2017;**2017**:3837194, 1-13. DOI: 10.1155/2017/3837194

[79] Ning Z, Lao L. Acupuncture for pain management in evidence-based

medicine. Journal of Acupuncture and Meridian Studies. 2015;**8**:270-273. DOI: 10.1016/J.JAMS.2015.07.012

[80] Chiu HY, Hsieh YJ, Tsai PS. Systematic review and meta-analysis of acupuncture to reduce cancer-related pain. European Journal of Cancer Care (Engl). 2017;**26**:e12457

[81] Lau CHY, Wu X, Chung VCH, et al. Acupuncture and related therapies for symptom management in palliative cancer care: Systematic review and meta-analysis. Medicine. 2016;**95**:1-13. Epub ahead of print 4 March 2016. DOI: 10.1097/MD.0000000000002901

[82] Casimiro L, Barnsley L, Brosseau L, Milne S, Welch V, Tugwell P, et al. Acupuncture and electroacupuncture for the treatment of rheumatoid arthritis. Cochrane Database of Systematic Reviews. 2005;(4):1-14. Art. No.: CD003788. DOI: 10.1002/14651858.cd003788.pub2

[83] Kwon YD, Pittler MH, Ernst E. Acupuncture for peripheral joint osteoarthritis: A systematic review and meta-analysis. Rheumatology. 2006;**45**:1331-1337

[84] Manheimer E, White A, Berman B, et al. Meta-analysis: Acupuncture for low back pain. Annals of Internal Medicine. 2005;**142**:651-663

[85] Cho YH, Kim CK, Heo KH, et al. Acupuncture for acute postoperative pain after back surgery: A systematic review and meta-analysis of randomized controlled trials. Pain Practice. 2015;**15**:279-291

[86] Lu Z, Dong H, Wang Q, et al. Perioperative acupuncture modulation: More than anaesthesia. BJA: British Journal of Anaesthesia. 2015;**115**:183-193

[87] Tola YO, Chow KM, Liang W. Effects of non-pharmacological interventions on preoperative anxiety and postoperative pain in patients undergoing breast cancer surgery: A systematic review. Journal of Clinical Nursing. 2021;**00**:1-16

[88] Ajorpaz NM, Mohammadi A, Najaran H, et al. Effect of music on postoperative pain in patients under open heart surgery. Nursing and Midwifery Studies. 2014;**3**:1-6

[89] Vaajoki A, Pietilä A-M, Kankkunen P, et al. Effects of listening to music on pain intensity and pain distress after surgery: An intervention. Journal of Clinical Nursing. 2012;**21**:708-717

[90] Dion L, Engen DJ, Lemaine V, et al. Massage therapy alone and in combination with meditation for breast cancer patients undergoing autologous tissue reconstruction: A randomized pilot study. Complementary Therapies in Clinical Practice. 2016;**23**:82-87

[91] Solaiman H, Mohamed S. Effects of Zikr meditation and jaw relaxation on postoperative pain, anxiety and physiologic response of patients undergoing abdominal surgery. Journal of Biology, Agriculture and Healthcare. 2013;**3**:23-38

[92] Franco L, Blanck TJJ, Dugan K, et al. Both lavender fleur oil and unscented oil aromatherapy reduce preoperative anxiety in breast surgery patients: A randomized trial. Journal of Clinical Anesthesia. 2016;**33**:243-249

[93] Beyliklioğlu A, Arslan S. Effect of lavender oil on the anxiety of patients before breast surgery. Journal of Perianesthesia Nursing. 2019;**34**:587-593

[94] Nilsson U. The anxiety- and pain-reducing effects of music interventions: A systematic review. AORN Journal.

2008;**87**. Epub ahead of print April 2008. DOI: 10.1016/j.aorn.2007.09.013

[95] Costa F, Ockelford A, Hargreaves DJ. The effect of regular listening to preferred music on pain, depression and anxiety in older care home residents. Psychology of Music. 2018;**46**:174-191

[96] Bae I, Lim HM, Hur MH, et al. Intra-operative music listening for anxiety, the BIS index, and the vital signs of patients undergoing regional anesthesia. Complementary Therapies in Medicine. 2014;**22**:251-257

[97] Emami ZA, Jafari H, Khani S, et al. The effect of music on the vital signs and SpO2 of patients after open heart surgery: A randomized clinical trial. Journal of Mazandaran University of Medical Sciences. 2011;**21**:73-82

[98] Sarıtaş SÇ, Araç B. The effect of music therapy on the vital signs of patients in a surgical intensive care unit. International Journal of Medical Investigation. 2016;**5**:54-59

[99] Zarurati M, Pishgooie SAH, Farsi Z, et al. The effect of music therapy on comfort level and some vital signs of patients undergoing hemodialysis. Military Caring Sciences. 2017;**3**:221-232

[100] Chlan LL. Music intervention. In: Snyder M, Lindquist R, editors. Complementary and Alternative Therapies in Nursing. New York, NY: Springer Publishing Company, LLC; 2018. pp. 91-105

[101] Finlay KA, Anil K. Passing the time when in pain: Investigating the role of musical valence. Psychomusicology: Music, Mind, and Brain. 2016;**26**:56-66

[102] Garza Villarreal EA, Brattico E, Vase L, et al. Superior analgesic effect of an active distraction versus pleasant unfamiliar sounds and music: The influence of emotion and cognitive style. PLoS One. 2012;**7**:1-8. Epub ahead of print 5 January 2012. DOI: 10.1371/JOURNAL.PONE.0029397

[103] Garcia RL, Hand CJ. Analgesic effects of self-chosen music type on cold pressor-induced pain: Motivating vs. relaxing music. Psychology of Music. 2016;**44**:967-983

[104] Basiński K, Zdun-Ryżewska A, Greenberg DM, et al. Preferred musical attribute dimensions underlie individual differences in music-induced analgesia. Scientific Reports. 2021;**11**:1-8. Epub ahead of print 1 December 2021. DOI: 10.1038/S41598-021-87943-Z

[105] Robb SL, Burns DS, Carpenter JS. Reporting guidelines for music-based interventions. Music Medicine. 2011;**3**:271-279

[106] Glasziou P. Music in hospital. The Lancet. 2015;**386**:1609-1610

[107] Wigram T, Pedersen IN, Bonde L. Models and methods of music therapy. A Comprehensive Guide to Music Therapy: Theory, Clinical Practice and Training. 2002:113-150

[108] Chanda ML, Levitin DJ. The neurochemistry of music. Trends in Cognitive Sciences. 2013;**17**:179-193

[109] Poulsen MJ, Coto J. Nursing music protocol and postoperative pain. Pain Management Nursing. 2018;**19**:172-176

[110] Finlay KA. Music-induced analgesia in chronic pain: Efficacy and assessment through a primary-task paradigm. Psychology of Music. 2014;**42**:325-346

[111] Bradt J, Potvin N, Kesslick A, et al. The impact of music therapy versus music medicine on psychological

outcomes and pain in cancer patients: A mixed methods study. Supportive Care in Cancer. 2015;**23**:1261-1271

[112] Bradt J, Dileo C, Shim M. Music interventions for preoperative anxiety. Cochrane Database of Systematic Reviews. 2013;**2013**. DOI: 10.1002/14651858.CD006908.pub2

[113] Fredenburg HA, Silverman MJ. Effects of music therapy on positive and negative affect and pain with hospitalized patients recovering from a blood and marrow transplant: A randomized effectiveness study. Arts in Psychotherapy. 2014;**41**:174-180

[114] Allred KD, Byers JF, Sole M, lou. The effect of music on postoperative pain and anxiety. Pain Management Nursing. 2010;**11**:15-25

[115] Greenlee H, DuPont-Reyes MJ, Balneaves LG, et al. Clinical practice guidelines on the evidence-based use of integrative therapies during and after breast cancer treatment. CA: A Cancer Journal for Clinicians. 2017;**67**:194-232

[116] Lowenstein KG. Meditation and self-regulatory techniques. In: Handbook of Complementary and Alternative Therapies in Mental Health. 2002. pp. 159-181. DOI: 10.1016/B978-012638281-5/50009-7

[117] Hofmann SG, Sawyer AT, Witt A, et al. Mindfulness for depression and anxiety. A meta-analysis. Journal Consulting Clinical Psychology. 2010;**78**:169-183

[118] Zeidan F, Martucci KT, Kraft RA, et al. Brain mechanisms supporting the modulation of pain by mindfulness meditation. Journal of Neuroscience. 2011;**31**:5540-5548

[119] Zeidan F, Martucci KT, Kraft RA, et al. Neural correlates of mindfulness meditation-related anxiety relief. Social Cognitive and Affective Neuroscience. 2014;**9**:751-759

[120] Sharon H, Maron-Katz A, ben Simon E, et al. Mindfulness meditation modulates pain through endogenous opioids. The American Journal of Medicine. 2016;**129**:755-758

[121] Kiran U, Ladha S, Makhija N, et al. The role of rajyoga meditation for modulation of anxiety and serum cortisol in patients undergoing coronary artery bypass surgery: A prospective randomized control study. Annals of Cardiac Anaesthesia. 2017;**20**:158

[122] Jinich-Diamant A, Garland E, Baumgartner J, et al. Neurophysiological mechanisms supporting mindfulness meditation–based pain relief: An updated review. Current Pain and Headache Reports. 2020;**24**:1-10

[123] Halcon LL. Aromatherapy. In: Lindquist R, Tracy MF, Snyder M, editors. Complementary and Alternative Therapies in Nursing. New York, NY: Springer Publishing Company, LLC; 2018

[124] Tamaki K, Fukuyama AK, Terukina S, et al. Randomized trial of aromatherapy versus conventional care for breast cancer patients during perioperative periods. Breast Cancer Research and Treatment. 2017;**162**:523-531

[125] d'Angelo R. Aromatherapy. Handbook of Complementary and Alternative Therapies in Mental Health. 2002:71-92

[126] Boehm K, Büssing A, Ostermann T. Aromatherapy as an adjuvant treatment in cancer care: A descriptive systematic review. African Journal of Traditional, Complementary, and Alternative Medicines. 2012;**9**:503-518

[127] Buckle J. Clinical Aromatherapy: Essential Oils in Healthcare. 3rd ed. Philadelphia: Churchill Livingstone; 2015

[128] Price S. Aromatherapy for Health Professionals. 2nd ed. Edinburgh: Churchill Livingstone; 1999

[129] Babashahi M, Fayazi S, Aghel N, et al. Effect of aromatherapy on anxiety level among preoperative patients. Jundishapur Scientific Medical Journal. 2010;**9**:507-516

[130] Buckle J. Stress and well-being. In: Clinical Aromatherapy: Essential of Oil in Healthcare. 3rd ed. Philadelphia: Churchill Livingston; 2015. pp. 223-237. DOI: 10.1016/B978-0-7020-5440-2.00011-5

[131] Wotman M, Levinger J, Leung L, et al. The efficacy of lavender aromatherapy in reducing preoperative anxiety in ambulatory surgery patients undergoing procedures in general otolaryngology. Laryngoscope Investig Otolaryngology. 2017;**2**:437-441

[132] Imanishi J, Kuriyama H, Shigemori I, et al. Anxiolytic effect of aromatherapy massage in patients with breast cancer. Evidence-based Complementary and Alternative Medicine. 2009;**6**:123-128

[133] Kim JT, Wajda M, Cuff G, et al. Evaluation of aromatherapy in treating postoperative pain: Pilot study. Pain Practice. 2006;**6**:273-277

[134] Lakhan SE, Sheafer H, Tepper D. The effectiveness of aromatherapy in reducing pain: A systematic review and meta-analysis. Pain Research and Treatment. 2016;**2016**:1-13. Epub ahead of print 2016. DOI: 10.1155/2016/8158693

[135] Xiao Y, Li L, Xie Y, et al. Effects of aroma therapy and music intervention on pain and anxious for breast cancer patients in the perioperative period. Zhong Nan Da Xue Xue Bao. Yi Xue Ban. 2018;**43**:656-661

[136] Ghavami H, Safarzadeh F, Asl RGA. Effect of self-care interventions on sleep quality in post-coronary artery bypass grafting patients: A single-center, randomized-controlled study. Turkish Journal of Thoracic and Cardiovascular Surgery. 2018;**26**:550-556

[137] Hashemzadeh K, Dehdilani M. The effect of aromatherapy on anxiety in patients before coronary artery bypass graft surgery. International Journal of New Chemistry. 2022;**9**:647-655

[138] Miozzo AP, Stein C, Bozzetto CB, et al. Massage therapy reduces pain and anxiety after cardiac surgery: A systematic review and meta-analysis of randomized clinical trials. Clinical Trials and Regulatory Science in Cardiology. 2016;**23-24**:1-8

[139] Snyder M, Taniguki S. Massage. In: Snyder M, Lindquist R, editors. Complementary and Alternative Therapies in Nursing. New York, NY: Springer Publishing Company, LLC; 2018

[140] Rosen J, Lawrence R, Bouchard M, et al. Massage for perioperative pain and anxiety in placement of vascular access devices. Advances in Mind—Body Medicine. 2013;**27**:12-23

[141] Dion L, Rodgers N, Cutshall SM, et al. Effect of massage on pain management for thoracic surgery patients. International Journal of Therapeutic Massage & Bodywork. 2011;**4**:2-6

[142] Massingill J, Jorgensen C, Dolata J, et al. Myofascial massage for chronic pain and decreased upper extremity mobility after breast cancer surgery. International Journal of Therapeutic Massage and

Bodywork: Research, Education, and Practice. 2018;**11**:4-9

[143] Wilson AT, Riley JL, Bishop MD, et al. A psychophysical study comparing massage to conditioned pain modulation: A single blind randomized controlled trial in healthy participants. Journal of Bodywork and Movement Therapies. 2021;**27**:426-435

[144] Sagar SM, Dryden T, Wong RK. Massage therapy for cancer patients: A reciprocal relationship between body and mind. Current Oncology. 2007;**14**:45-56

[145] Bauer BA, Cutshall SM, Wentworth LJ, et al. Effect of massage therapy on pain, anxiety, and tension after cardiac surgery: A randomized study. Complementary Therapies in Clinical Practice. 2010;**16**:70-75

[146] Albert NM, Gillinov AM, Lytle BW, et al. A randomized trial of massage therapy after heart surgery. Heart & Lung. 2009;**38**:480

[147] Chun-yan Y. Practice study on massage effects on stress response of patients awaiting cardiovascular surgery. Heart. 2011;**97**. Epub ahead of print October 2011. DOI: 10.1136/heartjnl-2011-300867.500

[148] Kaur S, Lobo DJ, Latha T. Role of foot and hand massage on the anxiety for postoperative open heart surgery patients: A randomized control trial. International Journal of Nursing Education. 2013;**5**:205-208

[149] Najafi SS, Rast F, Momennasab M, et al. The effect of massage therapy by patients' companions on severity of pain in the patients undergoing post coronary artery bypass graft surgery: A single-blind randomized clinical trial. International Journal of Community Based Nurs Midwifery. 2014;**2**:128-135

[150] Boitor M, Gélinas C, Richard-Lalonde M, et al. The effect of massage on acute postoperative pain in critically and acutely ill adults' post-thoracic surgery: Systematic review and meta-analysis of randomized controlled trials. Heart & Lung: The Journal of Acute and Critical Care. 2017;**46**:339-346

[151] Ucuzal M, Kanan N. Foot massage: Effectiveness on postoperative pain in breast surgery patients. Pain Management Nursing. 2014;**15**:458-465

[152] Asadizaker M, Fathizadeh A, Haidari A, et al. The effect of foot and hand massage on postoperative cardiac surgery pain. International Journal of Nursing and Midwifery. 2011;**3**:165-169

[153] Khalkhali H, Tanha ZER, Feizi A, et al. Effect of applying cold gel pack on the pain associated with deep breathing and coughing after open heart surgery. Iranian Journal of Nursing and Midwifery Research. 2014;**19**:545-549

[154] Ebrahimi-Rigi H, Feizi A, Abdollahimohammad A, et al. Effect of cold therapy on the pain of deep-breathing and coughing in patients after coronary artery bypass grafting. Der Pharmacia Lettre. 2016;**8**:201-205

[155] Ertuğ N, Ülker S. The effect of cold application on pain due to chest tube removal. Journal of Clinical Nursing. 2012;**21**:784-790

[156] Zencir G, Eser I. Effects of cold therapy on pain and breathing exercises among median sternotomy patients. Pain Management Nursing. 2016;**17**:401-410

[157] Johnson MI, Paley CA, Howe TE, Sluka KA. Transcutaneous electrical nerve stimulation for acute pain. Cochrane Database of Systematic Reviews. 2015. DOI: 10.1002/14651858.CD006142.pub3

[158] Jahangirifard A, Razavi M, Ahmadi ZH, et al. Effect of TENS on postoperative pain and pulmonary function in patients undergoing coronary artery bypass surgery. Pain Management Nursing. 2018;**19**:408-414

[159] Martínez-Rodríguez A, Senin-Camargo F, Raposo-Vidal I, et al. Effects of transcutaneous electrical nerve stimulation via peroneal nerve or soleus muscle on venous flow: A randomized cross-over study in healthy subjects. Medicine (United States). 2018;**97**. Epub ahead of print 1 September 2018. DOI: 10.1097/MD.0000000000012084

[160] Melzack R. The short-form McGill pain questionnaire. Pain. 1987;**30**:191-197. Available from: http://www.ncbi.nlm.nih.gov/pubmed/3670870

[161] Vance CGT, Dailey DL, Rakel BA, et al. Using TENS for pain control: The state of the evidence. Pain Management. 2014;**4**:197-209

Chapter 10

Postoperative Pain in Orthopedics

Lourdes Trinidad Castillo García,
Fabiola Estela Elizabeth Ortega Ponce
and Aurora Carolina Martínez Esparza

Abstract

Most patients who undergo orthopedic surgery experience moderate-to-severe discomfort. Historically, opioids have been the primary medication class used to treat pain transmission pathways. In orthopedic practice, multimodal analgesia has become the predominant method of pain management. Utilizing multiple medications to treat post-surgical pain reduces the need for narcotics and accelerates the healing process. By introducing effective analgesic treatments and interventions, this procedure reduces the use of perioperative opioids and, over time, the risk of opioid toxicity and addiction. Previous research has demonstrated that multimodal analgesia reduces the use of analgesics in the early postoperative period for orthopedic procedures. Numerous substances can stimulate or sensitize directly. When the peripheral nociceptors are damaged, direct damage to the nervous system results in pain. Preoperative, intraoperative, and postoperative symptoms are essential. The emphasis is on management regimes and the pathophysiology underlying the mechanism for postoperative discomfort. A concise description of the effects of painkillers is provided. containing information on specific conditions and average dosage substances are classified further. Both neuropathy and subjective pain should be treated. By focusing on multimodal analgesia, anesthesiologists can reduce pain more effectively. More advanced techniques are utilized for postoperative pain management after orthopedic surgery, thereby enhancing the patient's short- and long-term outcomes.

Keywords: orthopedic surgery, multimodal analgesia, pain management, anesthesiology, regional anesthesia, opioids

1. Introduction

One of the most painful operations a patient can have is orthopedic surgery.

Pain is defined as "A unpleasant sensory and emotional experience associated with, or resembling that associated with, actual or potential tissue damage" by the new International Association for the Study of Pain (IASP) definition. Most patients who undergo orthopedic surgery, particularly total joint replacement, experience moderate to severe pain.

One of the most significant developments in the field of total joint replacement surgery has been the improvement of pain management. In these patients, effective pain management speeds up recovery, accelerates healing, and enhances quality of

IntechOpen

life after surgery. According to the Joint Commission on Accreditation of Healthcare Organizations (JCAHO), pain has evolved into the "fifth vital sign" and must be taken into account when providing care for all patients. Throughout the entire inpatient and outpatient course, as well as when deciding whether to discharge a patient, pain must be taken into account. Pain must be treated, and failing to do so may result in medical malpractice claims. Since Professor Henrik Kehlet first proposed the idea of Enhanced Recovery After Surgery (ERAS), multimodal analgesia has gained popularity as a technique for treating pain. It requires for multidisciplinary cooperation between patients, doctors, anesthesiologists, physiotherapists, occupational therapists, and nursing staff and involves preoperative, perioperative, and postoperative components. When post-surgical pain is treated with multiple approaches, such as psychotherapy, physical therapy, regional anesthesia, local injections, and non-opioid medications, the recovery process is sped up, the need for opioids is reduced, and the risk of abuse is reduced. Multimodal analgesia has been proven in prior research to reduce both the length of stay and discomfort in the initial 24 hours following foot and ankle surgery. Opioid use was decreased postoperatively by combining periarticular injections with usual pain management for hip hemiarthroplasty. Injections at the surgical site for femur fracture and upper extremity surgeries reduced pain and raised overall patient satisfaction.

2. Incidence of pain

Postoperative pain is a common phenomenon after an orthopedic surgery and can be a limiting factor for the patient's recovery. The incidence of postoperative pain can vary depending on the type and technique of the surgery.

It is well known that the joint replacement surgery and spine surgery are the most painful surgeries, postoperative talking. In a multicenter study, by Arefaine [1] et al., in 2020, they found that moderate to severe postoperative pain was present in 70.5% of patients who underwent an orthopedic emergency surgery. They also found that orthopedics patients who had preoperative anxiety were 6.42 times more likely to develop moderate to severe postoperative pain compared with those patients who were not anxious, among other factors like history of preoperative anxiety, history of preoperative pain, preoperative patient expectation about postoperative pain, intraoperative use of tourniquet, type of anesthesia and duration of anesthesia were significant.

To handle the postoperative pain in an orthopedic surgery, several strategies have been used. One of the most common strategies is opioid use. However, some of the adverse effects they can cause nausea, vomit, sedation, and constipation. Also, opioid use can be addictive and increase it overdose use. Another strategy for an adequate postoperative pain management is the use of peripheral nerve blocks; studies demonstrated higher reported patient satisfaction of postoperative pain control in patients who received combined [2].

Peripheral nerve blocks (PNB) have remarkable benefits for immediate postoperative pain control after primary total hip arthroplasty (THA). The analgesic effect of PNB with IV PCA was better than conventional IV PCA alone [3].

Multimodal Analgesia (MMA), also referred to as "balanced analgesia," uses multiple analgesic medications, physical modalities, and cognitive strategies to affect peripheral and central nerve loci for the treatment of pain [4].

In regard of the technique, some studies found no significant difference in pain control, but they report significantly more effective in early mobilization with intraarticular infiltration [5].

2.1 Opioid overdose and addiction in the intrahospital setting

Opioid overdose and addiction are a common problem in the intrahospital setting, especially in patients who receive them for postoperative pain prolonged periods. Opioids are a class of analgesic that is highly effective and can be highly addictive and dangerous if wrongly used. According to a report from the CDC of the US, the rate of deaths for overdose use of opioids in the country went as high as 38% in 2019 and 2020, suggesting that the crisis is far from gone [6].

In the intrahospital setting, opioid overdose can occur as a result of an accidental or intentional overdose, or from an interaction with other medication. According to a study published in *JAMA Surgery Magazine*, 8.8% of patients that received opioids after a surgery developed addiction after 6 months [7]. In order to prevent overdose and addiction in the intrahospital setting, various strategies have been implemented. One of the most effective strategies is the protocol implementation for multimodal pain management, which imply the use of multiple analgesia modalities, like the peripheral nerve block and regional anesthesia [5]. They also implemented the use of short-action opioids and the reduction of prolonged-action opioids.

They have also implemented education and capacitation of medical and nurse professionals about the appropriate use of opioids and the early detection in its addiction, as well as the supervision of patients receiving opioids to detect early addiction or overdose signs. In conclusion, multimodal pain management protocol implementation, education and capacitation of medical and nurse professionals, and supervision are effective strategies for preventing these kinds of problems.

3. Postoperative pain in orthopedic surgery-associated factors

Postoperative pain is a common problem in orthopedic surgery and can have a meaningful impact on the patient's quality of life. There are several factors associated with postoperative pain in orthopedic surgery, including its severity, patient's age and anesthetic technique used. The severity of the surgery is an important factor that has been associated with postoperative pain, the more complex and invasive the surgery, for example, a total hip or knee arthroplasty, is associated with a higher incidence and severity of postoperative pain compared with simpler procedures like a fixed fracture [8]. Patient's age has also been related with postoperative pain in orthopedic surgery. Older patients can have less pain tolerance and can require an adequate strategy for its management [9, 10]. The anesthetic technique used can also be a part of the postoperative pain. Peripheral nerve blocks and regional anesthesia have been associated with a reduction in postoperative pain and opioid use [11, 12].

In order to prevent and handle postoperative pain in orthopedic surgery, various strategies have been implemented. One of the most effective strategies is the protocol implementation for multimodal pain management, which imply the use of multiple analgesia modalities to reduce the use of opioids and help in the patient's well-being [13]. They have also implemented patient's education about pain management and early mobilization [14].

In conclusion, postoperative pain is a common problem in orthopedic surgery and is associated to several factors like severity of the surgery, patient's age, and anesthetic technique used. Protocol implementation of multimodal pain management and patient's education are effective strategies for the reduction of postoperative pain.

4. ERAS protocol in orthopedic surgery

The ERAS Protocol (Enhanced Recovery After Surgery), is a multidisciplinary approach designed for the patient's recovery after surgery. This approach has been used widely in orthopedic surgery for the reduction in the intrahospital stay, postoperative pain, and opioid needs [15].

4.1 Components of enhanced recovery after surgery in orthopedic surgery

Preoperative interventions include patient's education about the recuperation process, nutrition and hydration, as well as respiratory and cardiovascular optimization. Intraoperative interventions include use of regional and multimodal anesthesia to reduce the necessity of opioids. Postoperative interventions include early mobilization, multimodal pain management and early hospital discharge [16].

The principal postoperative undesirable sequelae include pain, cardiopulmonary, infectious and thromboembolic complications, cerebral dysfunction, gastrointestinal paralysis, nausea, and prolonged hospital stay. Surgical and anesthetic techniques are related to the presence or severity in which the adverse effects can be present. On the other hand, one must consider changes related to organic function, which are present in every patient that goes through a surgical procedure, commonly known as surgical stress.

It has been proven that ERAS Protocol effectively reduces the length in intrahospital stay, postoperative pain and opioid need. It has also been demonstrated that the ERAS Protocol positively affects cardiopulmonary function, quality of life and patient's satisfaction [17]. However, implementation of the ERAS (**Tables 1** and **2**) Protocol in an orthopedic surgery can be quite challenging, as it requires an adequate collaboration between surgeons, anesthesiologists, nurses, and other healthcare specialists. Also, the ERAS Protocol implementation can require an expensive investment in resource and capacitation time.

ERAS In orthopedic surgery		
PREOPERATIVE Preoperative assessment and organ dysfunction optimization	**INTRAOPERATIVE** Stress-free anesthesia and surgery	**POSTOPERATIVE** Enhancing postoperative comfort and optimizing postoperative care
Optimize any organ dysfunction Optimize preoperative anemia Alcohol and smoking cessation education Fasting and nutrition Preoperative anesthetics and analgesics Prophylaxis against thromboembolism	Minimally invasive surgical techniques Anesthesia technique Local infiltration analgesia Maintaining normothermia Optimal intraoperative fluid balance Intraoperative anesthetics and analgesics Goal-directed fluid management	Multimodal opioid-sparing analgesic techniques Prevention of postoperative nausea and vomiting Early immobilization and rehabilitation

Table 1.
ERAS in orthopedic surgery.

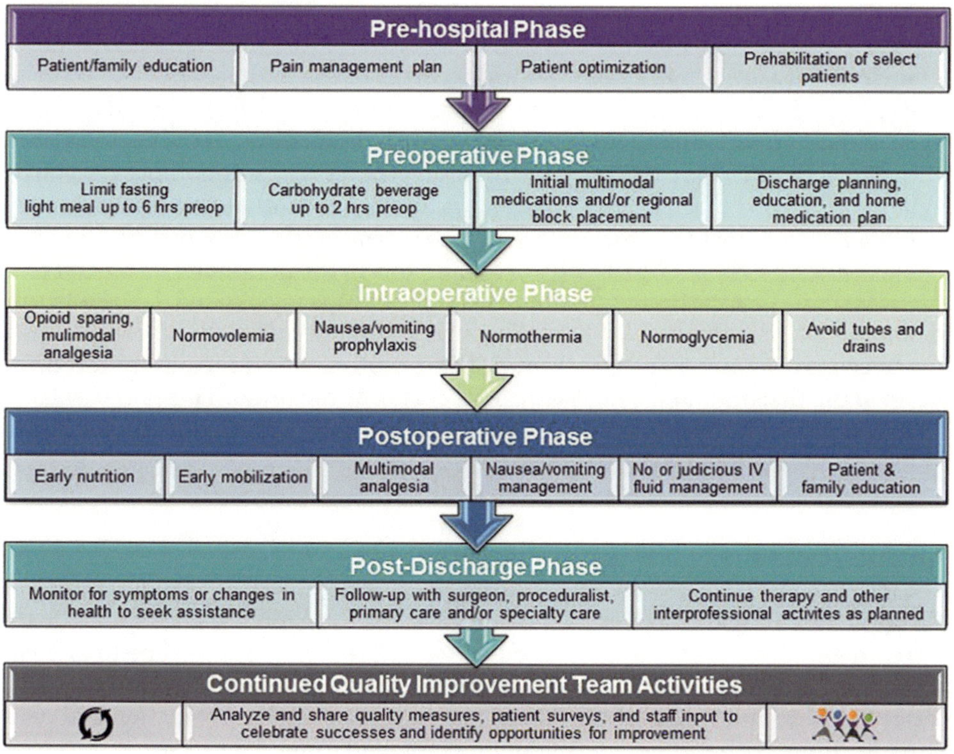

Table 2.
ERAS protocol implementation.

5. How does an inadequate treatment affect postoperative pain?

An inadequate treatment for postoperative pain can have a meaningful impact in a patient's recovery and his experience in his whole hospital stay. Uncontrolled pain can lead to anxiety, depression and prolonged hospital stay.

Postoperative pain is a common complication after surgery and can be caused by tissue damage, inflammation, and nerve manipulation. If not adequately controlled, pain can lead to a series of complications, like a prolonged hospital stay, greater risk of infection, and respiratory complications [18]. Pain can also affect quality of life, which can lead to a negative impact in patient's recuperation [19].

6. Pain's pathways

Pain is a complex complication that involves multiple pathways and systems in the human body. Knowledge of the different pathways of pain is fundamental for the development of effective therapeutic strategies to control it in different clinical conditions.

Somatic pathway of pain activates by painful stimuli that affect somatic tissue, like skin muscle, bone, and joints. This pathway transmits over nervous myelinated

A-Delta fibers and nervous non-myelinated C fibers. The information of this pathway is processed on the bone marrow and gets transmitted through the spinothalamic tract up to the thalamus and somatosensorial cortex of the brain [20].

Visceral pathway of pain activates by painful stimuli that affect internal organs, like the GI tract, heart, and lungs. This pathway transmits through the nervous non-myelinated C fibers. This pathway's information processes in autonomous nervous ganglia and the bone marrow, and it transmits through spinothalamic tract and the spinoreticular tract up to the thalamus and somatosensorial cortex of the brain [21].

Neuropathic pathway of pain activates by lesions in the peripheral or central nervous system. This pathway transmits through nervous myelinated A-Delta fibers and nervous non-myelinated C fibers, The information in this pathway gets processed in the bone marrow and transmits through the spinothalamic tract and spinoreticular tract up to the thalamus and somatosensorial cortex of the brain. This pathway is particularly difficult to treat because of the chronic nature of the pain and the lack of response to conventional analgesic medication [22].

7. Analgesic scale

World Health Organization (WHO) analgesic scale is a tool used for the evaluation and treatment of pain. This scale is based on pain classification according to intensity and the selection of an adequate analgesic for the treatment. In this section, it will be discussed the importance of the WHO analgesic scale for the evaluation and pain treatment, along with different levels and recommendations for its use.

The WHO Analgesic Scale is divided into four levels, according to the intensity of pain and the type of analgesic recommended for its treatment. The first level corresponds to a mild pain, and the recommendation is to use non-opioid analgesic, like acetaminophen or Ibuprofen. The second level corresponds to a moderate pain, and the recommendation is to use weak opioids, like codeine or tramadol. The third level corresponds to an intense pain, and the recommendation is to use strong opioids, like morphine or fentanyl. The fourth level corresponds to a refractory pain, and the recommendation is to use additional treatment, such as local anesthesia or nerve blocks [23].

The WHO analgesic scale is an important and useful tool used for the evaluation and treatment of pain, because it gives us a clear guidance for the selection of the analgesic according to the intensity of pain. Also, this scale helps professional healthcare workers to evaluate the efficacy of treatment of pain and make dose adjustments according to the patient's needs [24]. It is fundamental that this scale be used like a guidance and the treatment for pain must be individualized according to the needs of each patient. Professional healthcare workers must consider factors like age, comorbidities, individual sensibility and possible interaction with other medication [25].

8. Preventive analgesia

Focuses on postoperative pain control and the prevention of central sensitization and chronic neuropathic pain by providing analgesia administered preoperatively but not after surgical incision to reduce the intensity of postoperative pain [26]. Several studies have proven that preventive analgesia can aid postoperative analgesia and reduce the need of opioids after an orthopedic surgery. Preventive analgesia can also reduce inflammation and immune response, which can diminish the incidence of postoperative complications and shorten the patient's treatment [27].

The options for treatment of preventive analgesia in orthopedic surgery include the preoperative administration of pain medication, like NSAIDs, corticosteroids, and lidocaine, the use of regional anesthesia like nerve blocks, intraoperative administration of analgesics like opioids and local anesthetics [28]. In spite of all the benefits that preventive analgesia can provide in an orthopedic surgery, there are some challenges associated with its implementation. Dose selection and the moment of the administration can be hard to determine and can vary according to the type of orthopedic surgery. Also, preventive analgesia can be expensive and require a more complex monitoring during the surgery [29].

9. Pain evaluation

Pain evaluation is an important part of the treatment during an orthopedic surgery. Acute postoperative pain can be difficult to control and can have fatal consequences if not treated in time. The pain scale is a simple tool commonly used to evaluate postoperative pain. It asks the patient to rate their pain on a scale of 0–10, where 0 represents the absence of pain and 10 represents the worst imaginable pain. The pain scale is easy to evaluate and has been validated for its use in postsurgical patients [30].

Another tool commonly used to evaluate the pain is the Visual Analog Scale (VSA), which consists of a horizontal line of 10 cm, with the words "No Pain" on one end and "Worst Possible Pain" on the other end. Patients mark over the line to show the level of pain they are experiencing. This scale has demonstrated its valid and easy reproduction for the evaluation of postoperative pain [31].

Besides the pain scales, patients can describe pain using descriptive terms, such as "oppressive," "burn," "throbbing," or "colicky." The use of these words can help doctors to determine the pain's origin and choose the right treatment. In addition, the intensity of pain, a pain evaluation must include its location, duration, and effects on the physical function and quality of the patient's life. A pain evaluation must include the psychological and social factors that can relate to the perception of pain and its response to the treatment [32].

It is important to take into consideration that the pain evaluation is subjective, and it can be affected by cultural, social, or emotional factors, and that is why it is important to consider the experience and perspective of the patient in order to determine the postoperative pain in an orthopedic surgery.

10. Regional anesthesia

The control of postoperative pain is a crucial issue because its effectiveness will or may hamper early rehabilitation [33]. Richman and coworkers performed a meta-analysis, which included 19 articles enrolling 603 patients, related to postoperative analgesia with continuous peripheral nerve blocks and opioids. All articles showed that perineural analgesia provided significantly better postoperative analgesia compared with opioids [34]. Regional anesthesia is the most appropriate way to control postoperative pain. However, improvement in pain control after single-shot administration is limited to the first 24 postoperative hours. Therefore, it is not likely to significantly change outcome because early rehabilitation during the first 2–3 postoperative days is necessary to minimize the accumulation of small amounts of periarticular blood and edema, the first stages of joint stiffness [35].

Regional anesthesia can be broadly divided into two categories: neuraxial anesthesia [spinal, epidural, combined spinal epidural (CSE)], and peripheral nerve blocks (upper and lower extremity blocks).

10.1 Neuraxial anesthesia

Spinal anesthetic is a great choice for lower limb orthopedic surgery. Delay in ambulation due to lower limb muscular weakness, the risk of urine retention of up to 17%, and pain following block regression are all factors that limit the use of spinal anesthetic in the ambulatory context. It is critical to choose the right agent for ambulatory spinal anesthesia [36].

The technique of inserting a needle or a catheter between the vertebrae and administering drugs into the epidural (epidural anesthesia) or subarachnoid space (spinal anesthesia) is known as neuraxial anesthesia (NA). The spinal nerve root is the target of NA. LA with adjuncts such as preservative-free opioids are the most common medications injected neuraxially. NA is frequently utilized in abdominal and lower extremity surgery. The length of surgical incision and surgical manipulation determine the sensory level required for a certain surgery. T10 is required for total hip arthroplasty (THA), open reduction and internal fixation of the femur, and hip fractures, whereas L1 is required for knee surgeries [37]. Spinal anesthesia is normally given as a single injection, whereas epidural anesthesia is given through an indwelling catheter for continuous infusion.

The level of spinal blockade is determined by the overall dose of LA combination, the baricity of the injected solution, and the patient's position following the block. An epidural catheter allows for continuous drug infusion, extending the length of anesthesia. To avoid trauma to the termination of the conus medullaris, the spinal anesthetic needle is often inserted at the level of the L2–L3 interspace or below. The needle entry site for epidural anesthesia is determined by the extent of the dermatomes necessary for the treatment. It is frequently put in the mid to lower lumbar region for orthopedic surgeries. The volume of local anesthetic injected determines the degree of epidural blockade, whereas the concentration of the local anesthetic determines the density of the block. When compared to epidural anesthesia, spinal anesthesia results in a denser and more reliable block with a lower rate of block failure [38, 39].

10.2 Peripheral nerve blocks

PNB include injecting a LA solution to a single nerve or nerve bundle to create sensory and motor blocking of a specific body location. The LA prevents painful impulses from reaching the central nervous system. PNB can be used for anesthesia or analgesia after surgery. It is usually given as a single shot, although a continuous infusion catheter can be used to prolong the analgesic impact after surgery. PNB is usually performed under ultrasound guidance to limit the hazards of intraneural and intravascular LA injection, avoid peripheral nerve damage, and assure proper LA distribution for a successful block.

10.2.1 Blocks for upper extremity orthopedic procedures

Understanding upper extremity peripheral nerve blocking requires a thorough understanding of brachial plexus anatomy. The brachial plexus provides the majority of the upper extremity's muscular and cutaneous nerve supply. The brachial plexus is made up of five ventral nerve roots (rami) that give rise to trunks, divisions, cords, and terminal branches. The nerve roots join together to produce the upper, middle, and lower trunks. The three trunks divide into six divisions, which join to produce three cords: lateral, posterior, and medial cords. The terminal branches of the three cords feed the majority of the upper extremity nerves. Nerves that are not part of the brachial plexus augment the cutaneous area of the shoulder and upper arm. The superficial cervical plexus (C3–C4) innervates the superior portion of the shoulder via the supraclavicular nerve. Seventy percent of the sensory innervation to the shoulder comes from the superior trunk via the suprascapular nerve, with the C5 and C6 nerve roots contributing the most. The second thoracic nerve root innervates the axilla. The brachial plexus is restricted at four points: The interscalene block is used to connect roots and trunks, the supraclavicular block is used to connect trunks and divisions, the infraclavicular block is used to connect cords, and the axillary block is used to connect terminal branches [40]. The most frequently performed upper limb blocks are shown in **Table 3**.

10.2.1.1 Interscalene block

The interscalene block is conducted at the brachial plexus roots-trunks level. The interscalene block anesthetizes C5–C8, as well as the supraclavicular branches of the cervical plexus C3–C4, which supply the skin over the acromion and the clavicle. The inferior trunk (C8–T1) is frequently spared; this is known as ulnar sparing. As

Block	Clinical application	Nerves blocked	Anatomical landmarks	Complications
Interscalene nerve block	Surgeries involving the shoulder, proximal aspect of humerus, and the distal aspect of the clavicle	(1) Brachial plexus: C5 to C7 and (2) cervical plexus: supraclavicular nerve (C3 and C4)	LA injected between anterior and middle scalene muscles lateral to carotid artery and internal jugular vein	(1) Phrenic nerve palsy (100%); (2) Horner syndrome; and (3) Hoarseness
Supraclavicular nerve block	Surgery of the arm, elbow, forearm, and hand. Extension into the interscalene area can cover shoulder procedures	C5–T1	LA injected above the clavicle between anterior and middle scalene muscles at the level of the first rib, where the subclavian artery crosses over it	(1) Pneumothorax; (2) phrenic nerve palsy; and (3) hoarseness
Infraclavicular nerve block	Surgery of the elbow, forearm and hand	C5–T1	LA injected around the axillary artery below the clavicle, medial to coracoid process	Pneumothorax (relatively low incidence)
Axillary nerve block	Surgery of the elbow, forearm, and hand	Median nerve, ulnar nerve, radial nerve, and musculocutaneous nerve	LA injected around the axillary artery at the medial aspect of proximal arm	(1) Hematoma formation; and (2) intravascular injection

Table 3.
Upper extremity blocks.

a result, if this block is used for procedures at or near the elbow, an additional ulnar nerve block is required. This nerve block's coverage makes it useful for treatments involving the shoulder, proximal aspect of the humerus, and distal aspect of the clavicle [41].

The brachial plexus is targeted by the interscalene block, which is located lateral to the carotid artery and internal jugular vein, directly above the collarbone. Complications of the interscalene block include near-complete phrenic nerve blockade, sympathetic chain blockade resulting in Horner's syndrome, inadvertent injection in the vertebral artery, recurrent laryngeal nerve blockade resulting in hoarseness, and peripheral neuropathy. Pneumothorax, epidural injection, intrathecal injection resulting in total spinal anesthesia, spinal cord damage, and dorsal scapular or long thoracic nerve injury are also rare complications [42].

10.2.1.2 Supraclavicular block

The supraclavicular block targets the brachial plexus above the collarbone at the trunks and divisions. The C5–C7 distribution includes the more superficial and lateral branches that supply the shoulder, lateral aspect of the arm, and forearm, as well as the deeper and more medial dependent branches of C8 and T1 that supply the hand and medial aspect of the forearm. Adequate local anesthetic distribution in both locations is required for successful nerve block of the arm and hand. A local anesthetic is injected between the anterior and middle scalene muscles at the level of the first rib, where the subclavian artery passes posterior to the midpoint of the clavicle. Because all of the trunks and divisions of the brachial plexus are closely packed and may be anesthetized at this location, the supraclavicular block causes anesthesia of the upper limb, including the shoulder [41].

10.2.1.3 Infraclavicular block

The infraclavicular block impacts the brachial plexus at the level of the cords before the axillary and musculocutaneous nerves branch. It causes numbness in the upper limb below the shoulder, including the arm, elbow, forearm, and hand, while leaving the medial proximal upper arm, which is supplied by the intercostobrachial nerve (T2), unaffected [42].

The infraclavicular block is injecting local anesthetic around the axillary artery beneath the clavicle. Under ultrasound guidance, the local anesthetic is administered in a U-shaped pattern around the axillary artery, encompassing all three brachial plexus cords. The infraclavicular block has a low pneumothorax rate of 0.7% [43].

10.2.1.4 Axillary block

The axillary block is performed at the level of the brachial plexus branches. It anesthetizes the median nerve, the ulnar nerve, the radial nerve, and the musculocutaneous nerve, resulting in upper limb numbness from the mid-arm to the elbow, forearm, and hand. It should be noted that this block does not obstruct the axillary nerve; rather, the term of this regional treatment comes from the approach. The patient is positioned supine with the arm abducted to 90° in order to conduct this block. The median, ulnar, and radial nerves are identified as they surround the axillary artery using ultrasound guidance [44].

10.2.2 Lower extremity peripheral nerve blocks

Peripheral nerve blocks can be used as a primary anesthetic modality or as a supplement to general or neuraxial anesthesia. Lower extremity nerve blocks are commonly used as an adjuvant to general or neuraxial anesthesia due to anatomical restrictions in attaining appropriate surgical anesthesia by peripheral nerve blockade [45]. The most frequently performed lower limb blocks are shown in **Table 4**.

10.2.2.1 Femoral nerve block

The femoral nerve block is used for lower extremity procedures that involve the anterior thigh and the medial side of the leg below the knee. The femoral nerve block is commonly used to provide analgesia for TKA, anterior cruciate ligament restoration, quadriceps tendon repair, foot surgery, and ankle surgery. The femoral nerve block can be coupled with other regional anesthetic methods, such as the sciatic nerve block, to broaden the anesthetic block's distribution, especially below the knee [46].

The femoral nerve provides sensory innervation to the anterior thigh and medial aspects of the calf, foot, and ankle. The femoral nerve additionally provides motor

Block	Clinical application	Nerves blocked	Anatomical landmarks	Complications
Femoral nerve (Femoral nerve block)	Surgeries involving anterior aspect of the thigh and medial aspect of the leg below the knee	Femoral nerve	Inguinal crease; located lateral to femoral artery	(1) LE weakness and falls; (2) bleeding; (3) infection; and (4) nerve damage
Femoral nerve (Fascia Iliaca block)	Surgeries involving anterior aspect of the thigh and medial aspect of the leg below the knee	(1) Femoral nerve and (2) lateral femoral cutaneous nerve of the thigh	Inguinal crease, LA injected under fascia iliaca	(1) LE weakness and falls; (2) bleeding; (3) infection; and (4) nerve damage
Sciatic nerve (Popliteal Block)	Surgeries involving foot, ankle, posterior knee	Sciatic nerve	Popliteal fossa, located cephalad to the knee near popliteal artery	Motor blockade
Saphenous nerve (Adductor Canal block)	Surgeries involving medial aspect of knee, foot, and ankle	(1) Saphenous nerve and (2) nerve to vastus medialis (branch of femoral nerve)	Medial thigh, located deep to the sartorius muscle, adjacent to the femoral artery and vein	(1) Bleeding; (2) infection; (3) nerve damage; and (4) potential lower extremity weakness at high doses
iPACK	Surgeries involving the posterior knee capsule	Articular branches of the tibial, common peroneal, and obturator nerve to the posterior aspect of the knee	Popliteal crease, located cephalad to femoral condyles	Inadvertent motor block due to local anesthetic spread to sciatic nerve branches

Table 4.
Lower extremity blocks.

innervation to muscles of the lower extremity, including the quadriceps, sartorius, and pectineus muscles. As such, the femoral nerve block will cause weakness of the quadriceps muscles [46, 47]. This may result in decreased patient mobility and may potentially increase the risk of falls. Thus, patients should not be ambulating without assistance after a femoral nerve block [47].

10.2.2.2 Iliac fascia block

The femoral nerve and lateral femoral cutaneous nerve are both anesthetized using the fascia iliac block, a regional anesthetic technique. It is used for analgesia following hip surgery or in people who have had catastrophic hip fractures. This block has been found to provide fast analgesic benefit and may be administered pre-operatively while the patient is waiting for their procedure. Additionally, patients reported gains from passive hip flexion, which enabled them to sit up in bed before surgery [48]. A shorter hospital stays, less discomfort, and a shorter time to fascia iliac block have all been linked to patients with hip fractures. When presented to the emergency room, a fascia iliac block can be performed, and research has shown that this block provides better pain relief than systemic intravenous opioid therapy. The fascia iliac block may also help these patients be positioned in the best way possible for the implantation of spinal anesthesia during surgical femur fracture repair [48, 49].

A rather significant volume of local anesthetic (20–30 cc) is injected under the fascia iliac, just above the level of the inguinal crease, to conduct the fascia iliac block. The purpose of this block, which is normally carried out under ultrasound guidance, is to disseminate local anesthetic medially to the femoral nerve and laterally to the iliac spine [50].

10.2.2.3 Adductor canal block

The adductor canal block effectively relieves pain during knee and medial lower limb surgery. For patients receiving TKA, it may be administered as a component of a multimodal analgesic pathway to promote early ambulation, enhance patient comfort, and boost patient satisfaction [51]. A majority of TKA patients will probably feel moderate-to-severe post-operative pain, which can lengthen recovery times, cause problems from immobility, and reduce patient satisfaction [52]. Therefore, for these patients, safe and efficient localized anesthetic procedures are crucial.

While the femoral nerve block can effectively reduce pain for patients having a complete knee replacement, it can also cause quadriceps muscle weakness, which may make a patient more likely to fall. Because of this, patients having TKR frequently find the adductor canal block to be a good choice for post-operative analgesia. The adductor canal block produces comparable levels of postoperative pain alleviation as the femoral nerve block while greatly sparing the quadriceps and preserving balance. This enables efficient pain management and the ability to encourage early mobilization and ambulation following surgery [53, 54]. The adductor canal block has widely become the standard of care for analgesia for total knee arthroplasty.

10.2.2.4 iPACK block

The iPACK block has been used more frequently in TKA to relieve pain without sacrificing the strength of the lower extremities in the posterior compartment of the knee. To effectively relieve pain in the posterior knee capsule, it targets the medial and lateral superior genicular nerves [55]. By guaranteeing coverage of both the antero-medial and posterior joints, the iPACK block and ACB together give a wider distribution of anesthetic coverage [55, 56].

According to recent research, the iPACK block, when combined with the adductor canal block and periarticular injection for TKA, significantly reduced postoperative pain during rest and ambulation [56, 57]. Early hospital discharge, a reduction in the need for opioids, and quicker ambulation were the outcomes.

Under ultrasound guidance, a needle is injected into the medial thigh to perform an iPACK block. This block typically uses a total volume of 15–20 cc of a local anesthetic solution. It is crucial to prevent accidental local anesthetic diffusion to the tibial or common peroneal nerve during the execution of this block, which could cause unfavorable motor weakness [58].

10.2.2.5 Sciatic nerve block

For lower extremity orthopedic procedures involving the foot, ankle, and posterior knee, a sciatic nerve block is indicated. The sciatic nerve block can be used alone, as in an Achilles tendon repair, or in conjunction with the femoral or saphenous nerve blocks to provide anesthetic coverage for knee surgery or foot/ankle surgery, respectively [59]. The sciatic nerve is the biggest nerve in the body, running from the anterior rami of L4 to S3. The tibial nerve and common peroneal nerve are the sciatic nerve's terminal branches. With the exception of the medial lower leg and foot, which is supplied by the saphenous nerve, the sciatic nerve block delivers analgesia to the posterior portion of the knee, hamstrings, and the entire limb below the knee (motor and sensory innervation).

Depending on the region of the limb requiring anesthetic blockade, the sciatic nerve may be blocked in numerous locations. The sciatic nerve block is administered on the proximal medial thigh via the anterior route. The transgluteal approach is used on the back of the buttock, between the ischial tuberosity and the greater trochanter. The subgluteal approach is conducted on the gluteal crease from the back. The sciatic nerve block is commonly administered at the level of the popliteal fossa, sometimes known as the "popliteal block" [59].

10.2.2.6 Popliteal block

For foot and ankle surgery, the popliteal nerve block is used in conjunction with the saphenous nerve block. The popliteal fossa is where the sciatic nerve splits into two major terminal branches, the tibial nerve and the common peroneal nerve [45]. A popliteal block is commonly performed proximal to the bifurcation of the tibial and common peroneal nerves; however, a recent study suggests that a popliteal block performed distal to the sciatic nerve bifurcation may result in a 30% faster onset of blockade while still achieving terminal branch blockade [59]. Furthermore, injection of local anesthetic distal to the sciatic nerve bifurcation offers better sensory block of the lower extremity.

Nerve damage, hemorrhage, and intravascular injection are all possible consequences of a sciatic nerve block. Nerve damage can cause a chronic foot drop with possible pressure necrosis [45, 60].

11. Regional anesthesia in patients at risk of bleeding

There have been no prospective studies on peripheral nerve blocks in the presence of anticoagulants. The ASRA recommends the same guidelines for peripheral nerve blocks as for neuraxial procedures. Cases of psoas and retroperitoneal hematomas have been reported after lumbar plexus nerve blocks and psoas compartment nerve blocks. These patients were either on enoxaparin, ticlopidine, or clopidogrel. In some cases, the hematoma occurred in spite of adherence to the ASRA guidelines.

It is probably too restrictive to adapt the ASRA guidelines on neuraxial nerve blocks to patients undergoing peripheral nerve blocks. The European Society of Anesthesiology has noted that the guidelines for neuraxial nerve block do not routinely apply to peripheral nerve blocks. The Austrian Society of Anesthesiology, Resuscitation and Intensive Care, on the other hand, has suggested that superficial nerve blocks can be safely performed in the presence of anticoagulants. Because of the possibility of retroperitoneal hematoma, lumbar plexus and paravertebral nerve blocks merit the same recommendations as for neuraxial injections. The same guidelines should also apply to visceral sympathetic nerve blocks. The ASRA guidelines may, therefore, be applicable to nerve blocks in vascular and noncompressible areas, such as a celiac plexus nerve blocks, superior hypogastric plexus nerve blocks, and lumbar plexus nerve blocks [61].

12. Nonsteroidal anti-inflammatory drugs

The mechanism of NSAIDs (nonsteroidal anti-inflammatory drugs) not only has been described by the peripheral inhibition of prostaglandin synthesis but also through a variety of other peripheral and central mechanism. The central role that augments its known peripheral action, by which it promotes the production of endogenous opioid peptides [62].

The healing process of fractures is a complex process which includes a combination of sequential set of events that depends on the stability of the fracture. There are many factors that influence this process, including the use of NSAIDs. The use of NSAIDs has been studied for many years with debatable effects on bone healing. Humaid Al Farii et al conclude from his meta-analysis that NSAIDs that do not include indomethacin can be used for pain management without having a significant effect on bone healing and additionally, the use of NSAIDs for short duration, less tan2 weeks, does not show a statistical in nonunion [63].

NSAIDS are proven to be effective for musculoskeletal pain, with head-to-head clinical studies noting equivalent pain control with NSAIDs compared with opioids with a reduced risk profile. Contraindications with NSAIDs include peptic ulcer disease, chronic or end-stage renal disease, bronchial asthma, and breastfeeding women [64].

12.1 Acetaminophen

Like NDSAIDS acetaminophen may be used after surgery to reduce the amount of stronger, opioid medications you need to control pain. Acetaminophen does not interfere with the COX-1 or COX-2 enzyme to reduce pain, so does not have anti-inflammatory properties. Used alone, Works well for headaches, fever, and minor aches and pains, but does not reduce the inflammation and swelling that might accompany a muscle sprain.

13. Opioids

13.1 Tramadol

Tramadol is a synthetic, centrally acting analgesic agent with 2 distinct but complementary mechanisms of action: selectivity for μ receptor, although it binds weakly to the δ and κ receptors. The affinity for the μ receptor is ≈6000 fold less than morphine and 10-fold less than codeine. Inhibits reuptake of noradrenaline (norepinephrine) and 5-HT. Causes no clinically relevant respiratory depression in adults or children undergoing surgery and there are no clinically significant changes in oxygen saturation in adults and children receiving tramadol. In healthy adult volunteers and patients who underwent abdominal surgery, tramadol had no clinically relevant effects on gastrointestinal functioning [65].

Three studies evaluated the effects of tramadol on postoperative pain, opioid consumption, and complications after primary total joint arthroplasty (TJA). One high quality study compared the use of tramadol versus a placebo for treatment of pain after TJA. Another high-quality study compared tramadol to placebo and to paracetamol with codeine. One additional high-quality study compared tramadol to other opioid medications for treatment of pain after TJA. There were mixed results among all studies on the effects of tramadol on pain, patient-reported outcome scores, opioid consumption and adverse events after TJA. Adverse events including dizziness, dry mouth, and nausea were more common among patients who received tramadol compared to placebo. Given the conflicting evidence with regards to opioid consumption, the fact that two studies evaluated intravenous tramadol which is not approved by the Food and Drug Administration in the United States, and that there was inconclusive evidence comparing the efficacy of tramadol to other opioids the strength of the recommendation was downgraded to moderate [66–68].

13.2 Morphine

Immediate release opioids are preferred in the management of postoperative pain when simple analgesics are insufficient to achieve the analgesic goals. If modified-release opioid preparations (including transdermal) are used, due care should be exercised as they have been associated with harm. The prescribed dose of the immediate release opioids should be age related (rather than weight) and take into account renal function. Immediate-release oxycodone is not recommended as a first line opioid, because is more labor intensive to administer. However, it is recognized that in elderly patients over 70 years or in patients with renal failure, other opioids may be used post operatively [69].

13.3 Oxycodone

Oxycodone is a semisynthetic, μ-opioid receptor agonist with analgesic effects in several pain conditions. Acts also on κ-opioid receptors. Oxycodone and morphine are presumed to have a 1:1 ratio of analgesic potency in postoperative pain after surgery, with mixed somatic and visceral pain components. Oxycodone is metabolized by the cytochrome P450 enzyme system in the liver [70]. Shows the same adverse effects as those typically found for opioids, with constipation (25–30%), nausea (25–30%), and drowsiness (25%) being the three most common symptoms. Vomiting, pruritus, and dizziness occur in 5%–15% of patients taking oxycodone [71]. The potency ratio of oxycodone to fentanyl is less than 75:1. It is necessary to reduce the analgesic dose of oxycodone in elderly patients because metabolic clearance decreases with age.

Oxycodone for somatic pain such as pain after orthopedic surgery, the amount of oxycodone should be higher than the dose used for visceral pain. In a study of seventy-three patients undergoing orthopedic surgery randomly assigned to receive fentanyl or oxycodone using intravenous PCA, they concluded that with a 1:60 ratio of oxycodone to fentanyl in the application of PCA for pain control, the use of larger doses of oxycodone for 6 hours is effective in controlling early postoperative pain [72].

13.4 Transdermal buprenorphine

It is more described for chronic pain management, that persists for 12 weeks or more despite analgesia [73]. The role in the clinical management for acute pain is less clear, but it has been evaluated in the postoperative setting of hip fracture surgery, knee or hip arthroscopy/arthroplasty, shoulder surgery and spinal surgery. Is a partial agonist at the μ-opioid receptor [74, 75]. When the patch is applied prior to surgery and left in place for the prescribed seven days, it is associated with reduce postoperative pian, lower consumption of other analgesics, and patient satisfaction.

Is an opioid and a Schedule III controlled substance which means it is considered less dangerous tan Schedule II substances, such as morphine or oxycodone [76]. Buprenorphine has a ceiling effect for respiratory depression, meaning that the risk for opioid-induce respiratory depression does not increase beyond a certain dose. Has hepatic metabolization, it is safe for patients with renal dysfunction. This means buprenorphine can be administered to elderly patients and those with renal dysfunction without the need to adjust the dose [77].

The transdermal buprenorphine patch is available in 5, 10 and 20 μg/h doses and other doses can be achieved by cutting the patch or using two patches. The transdermal buprenorphine patch is to be discontinued after seven days with the plan of switching the patient to an oral opioid or some other pain reliever, it is recommended that the buprenorphine patch be removed and 24 hours elapse before the new medication is started. Based on recent clinical trials, buprenorphine is 75–100 times more potent than morphine [78].

14. Conclusion

Any general or regional anesthetic technique must always be tailored to the individual patient and the procedure, taking the potential benefits and risks into account. The contribution of the individual anesthesiologist in managing the RA or GA (regional anesthesia or general anesthesia) technique effectively and safely in order to obtain a positive outcome should not be undervalued. In spite of this, evidence suggests that RA confers additional benefits beyond the reduction of acute pain. These include a distinct reduction in pulmonary complications and a reduction in chronic pain after certain procedures. RA has also been associated with a reduction in cancer recurrence, blood transfusion, severe sepsis, intensive care unit admissions, and even a small reduction in mortality in some cases; however, these findings should be interpreted with greater caution. When CNB (central neuraxial blockade) is administered alone, as opposed to in conjunction with GA, the benefits are frequently greater. Logically, utilizing PNBs without GA and thereby avoiding CNB-mediated hypotension may offer the greatest benefit; however, the potential outcome advantages of PNBs are the area that has received the least amount of research.

Definitely postoperative pain can have a significative impact in the physiology of the body, including the activation of inflammatory mediators and changes in cardiovascular, respiratory and GI function. The understanding of these physiological alterations is of vital importance for the correct treatment of postoperative pain and possible postoperative complications.

Conflict of interest

The authors declare no conflict of interest.

Notes/thanks/other declarations

None.

Author details

Lourdes Trinidad Castillo García*, Fabiola Estela Elizabeth Ortega Ponce and Aurora Carolina Martínez Esparza
Department of Anesthesia and Perioperative Pain, American British Cowdray Medical Center, Mexico City

*Address all correspondence to: lulucastillogarcia@gmail.com

References

[1] Arefayne NR, Tegegne SS, Gebregzi AH, Mustofa SY. Incidence and associated factors of post-operative pain after emergency Orthopedic surgery: A multi-centered prospective observational cohort study. International Journal of Surgery Open. 2020;**27**:103-113. DOI: doi.org/10.1016/j.ijso.2020.10.003

[2] Gianakos AL, Romanelli F, Rao N, Badri M, Lubberts B, et al. Combination lower extremity nerve blocks and their effect on postoperative pain and opioid consumption: A systematic review. The Journal of Foot and Ankle Surgery. 2021;**60**(1):121-131

[3] Park HJ, Park KK, Park JY, Lee B, Choi YS, Kwon HM. Peripheral nerve block for pain management after total hip arthroplasty: A retrospective study with propensity score matching. Journal of Clinical Medicine. 2022;**11**(18):5456. DOI: 10.3390/jcm11185456 PMID: 36143103; PMCID: PMC9505421

[4] Sampognaro G, Harrell R. Multimodal postoperative pain control after orthopaedic surgery. 2023. In: StatPearls [Internet]. Treasure Island, FL: StatPearls Publishing. PMID: 34283438.

[5] Karpetas GZ, Spyraki MK, Giakoumakis SI, Fligou FG, Megas PD, Voyagis GS, et al. Multimodal analgesia protocol for pain management after total knee arthroplasty: Comparison of three different regional analgesic techniques. Journal of Musculoskeletal & Neuronal Interactions. 2021;**21**(1):104-112 PMID: 33657760; PMCID: PMC8020020

[6] Centers for Disease Control and Prevention. Drug overdose deaths. (2021). Available from: https://www.cdc.gov/drugoverdose/deaths/index.html

[7] Brat GA, Agniel D, Beam A, Yorkgitis B, Bicket M, Homer M, et al. Postsurgical prescriptions for opioid naive patients and association with overdose and misuse: Retrospective cohort study. BMJ. 17 Jan 2018;**360**:j5790. DOI: 10.1136/bmj.j5790. PMID: 29343479; PMCID: PMC5769574

[8] Ljungqvist O, Scott M, Fearon KC. Enhanced recovery after surgery: A review. JAMA Surgery. 2017;**152**(3):292-298. DOI: 10.1001/jamasurg.2016.4952

[9] Yang Y, Chen S, Li K, et al. Enhanced recovery after surgery (ERAS) in total hip arthroplasty: A systematic review and meta-analysis. The Journal of Arthroplasty. 2020;**35**(7):1965-1973.e6. DOI: 10.1016/j.arth.2020.02.068

[10] Grant MC, Yang D, Wu CL, Makary MA, Wick EC. Impact of enhanced recovery after surgery and fast track surgery pathways on healthcare-associated in.

[11] Apfelbaum JL, Chen C, Mehta SS, Gan TJ. Postoperative pain experience: Results from a national survey suggest postoperative pain continues to be undermanaged. Anesthesia and Analgesia. 2003;**97**:534-540

[12] Wylde V, Rooker J, Halliday L, Blom AW. Acute postoperative pain at rest after hip and knee arthroplasty: Severity, sensory qualities and impact on sleep. Orthopaedics & Traumatology: Surgery & Research: OTSR. 2011;**97**:139-144

[13] Memtsoudis SG, Poeran J, Cozowicz C, et al. The impact of regional anesthesia on long-term survival after total knee arthroplasty: A population-based cohort analysis. Anesthesiology. 2018;**129**:225-235

[14] Joshi GP, Kehlet H. Multimodal analgesia techniques and postoperative rehabilitation. Anesthesiology Clinics. 2005;**23**(1):P185-P202. DOI: 10.1016/j.atc.2004.11.010

[15] Kehlet H. Multimodal approach to control postoperative pathophysiology and rehabilitation. British Journal of Anaesthesia. 1997;**78**:606-617

[16] Halawi MJ, Grant SA, Bolognesi MP. Multimodal analgesia for total joint arthroplasty. Orthopedics. 2015;**38**:e616

[17] McLeod RS, Aarts MA, Chung F, Eskicioglu C, Forbes SS, Conn LG, et al. Development of an enhanced recovery after surgery guideline and implementation strategy based on the knowledge-to-action cycle. Annals of Surgery. Dec 2015;**262**(6):1016-1025. DOI: 10.1097/SLA.0000000000001067. PMID: 25692358

[18] Kehlet H, Jensen TS, Woolf CJ. Persistent postsurgical pain: Risk factors and prevention. Lancet. 2006;**367**(9522):1618-1625. DOI: 10.1016/S0140-6736(06)68700-X

[19] Clark C, Curry CS. Postoperative pain management: A survey of patients' self-reported experiences. Journal of Pain Research. 2014;7:515-523. DOI: 10.2147/JPR.S63762

[20] Basbaum AI, Bautista DM, Scherrer G, Julius D. Cellular and molecular mechanisms of pain. Cell. 2009;**139**(2):267-284. DOI: 10.1016/j.cell.2009.09.028

[21] Merskey H, Bogduk N. Classification of Chronic Pain. IASP Task Force on Taxonomy. 2nd ed. Seattle: IASP Press; 1994. Available from: http://www.iasp-pain.org/Education/content.aspx?ItemNumber=1698

[22] Woolf CJ. Pain: Moving from symptom control toward mechanism-specific pharmacologic management. Annals of Internal Medicine. 2004;**140**(6):441-451. DOI: 10.7326/0003-4819-140-6-200403160-00010

[23] World Health Organization. Cancer pain relief and palliative care. Technical Report Series, No. 804. Geneva: World Health Organization; 1990.

[24] Carr DB, Jacox AK, Chapman CR, et al. Acute Pain Management: Operative or Medical Procedures and Trauma. Clinical practice guideline No. 1. AHCPR publication No. 92-0032. Rockville, MD: Agency for Health Care Policy and Research, Public Health Service, U.S. Department of Health and Human Services; 1992

[25] Mercadante S. Principles of opioid therapy in cancer pain. Journal of Clinical Oncology. 2014;**32**(16):1662-1670. DOI: 10.1200/JCO.2013.50.7894

[26] Vadivelu N, Mitra S, Schermer E, Kodumudi V, Kaye AD, Urman RD. Preventive analgesia for postoperative pain control: A broader concept. Local and Regional Anesthesia. 2014;**29**(7):17-22

[27] Weibel S, Jokinen J, Pace NL, et al. Efficacy and safety of acetaminophen, ibuprofen, and naproxen sodium for pain relief after ambulatory surgery: A randomized clinical trial. Anesthesiology. 2019;**131**(2):281-293. DOI: 10

[28] Lee IW, Schraag S. The use of intravenous lidocaine in perioperative medicine: Anaesthetic, analgesic and immune-modulatory aspects. Journal of Clinical Medicine. 2022;**11**(12):3543. DOI: 10.3390/jcm11123543 PMID: 35743617; PMCID: PMC9224677

[29] Wang D, Liu Z, Zhou J, Yang J, Chen X, Chang C, et al. Barriers to implementation of enhanced recovery after surgery (ERAS) by a

multidisciplinary team in China: A multicentre qualitative study. BMJ Open. 2022;**12**(3):e053687. DOI: 10.1136/bmjopen-2021-053687 PMID: 35288383; PMCID: PMC8921855

[30] Bijur PE, Silver W, Gallagher EJ. Reliability of the visual analog scale for measurement of acute pain. Academic Emergency Medicine. 2001;**8**(12):1153-1157

[31] Myles PS, Myles DB, Galagher W, Boyd D, Chew C, MacDonald N, et al. Measuring acute postoperative pain using the visual analog scale: The minimal clinically important difference and patient acceptable symptom state. British Journal of Anaesthesia. 2017;**118**(3):424-429. DOI: 10.1093/bja/aew466 PMID: 28186223

[32] Sierżantowicz R, Lewko J, Bitiucka D, Lewko K, Misiak B, Ładny JR. Evaluation of pain management after surgery: An observational study. Medicina (Kaunas, Lithuania). 2020;**56**(2):65. DOI: 10.3390/medicina56020065 PMID: 32046199; PMCID: PMC7073849

[33] Brown AR, Weiss R, Greenberg C, et al. Interscalene block for shoulder arthroscopy: Comparison with general anesthesia. Arthroscopy. 1993;**9**:295-300

[34] Richman JM, Liu SS, Courpas G, et al. Does continuous peripheral nerve block provide superior pain control to opioids? A meta-analysis. Anesthesia and Analgesia. 2006;**102**:248-257

[35] O'Driscoll SW, Giori NJ. Continuous passive motion (CPM): Theory and principles of clinical application. Journal of Rehabilitation Research and Development. 2000;**37**:179-188

[36] Imarengiaye CO, Song D, Prabhu AJ, et al. Spinal anesthesia: Functional balance is impaired after clinical recovery. Anesthesiology. 2003;**98**:511-515

[37] Carpenter RL, Caplan RA, Brown DL, Stephenson C, Wu R. Incidence and risk factors for side effects of spinal anesthesia. Anesthesiology. 1992;**76**:906-916 PMID: 1599111. DOI: 10.1097/00000542-199206000-00006

[38] Memtsoudis SG, Sun X, Chiu YL, Stundner O, Liu SS, Banerjee S, et al. Perioperative comparative effectiveness of anesthetic technique in orthopedic patients. Anesthesiology. 2013;**118**:1046-1058 PMID: 23612126. DOI: 10.1097/ALN.0b013e318286061d

[39] Pugely AJ, Martin CT, Gao Y, Mendoza-Lattes S, Callaghan JJ. Differences in short-term complications between spinal and general anesthesia for primary total knee arthroplasty. The Journal of Bone and Joint Surgery. American Volume. 2013;**95**:193-199 PMID: 23269359. DOI: 10.2106/JBJS.K.01682

[40] Bruce BG, Green A, Blaine TA, Wesner LV. Brachial plexus blocks for upper extremity orthopaedic surgery. The Journal of the American Academy of Orthopaedic Surgeons. 2012;**20**:38-47 PMID: 22207517. DOI: 10.5435/JAAOS-20-01-038

[41] Srikumaran U, Stein BE, Tan EW, Freehill MT, Wilckens JH. Upper-extremity peripheral nerve blocks in the perioperative pain management of orthopaedic patients: AAOS exhibit selection. The Journal of Bone and Joint Surgery. American Volume. 2013;**95**:e197 PMID: 24352782. DOI: 10.2106/JBJS.L.01745

[42] Melton MS, Monroe HE, Qi W, Lewis SL, Nielsen KC, Klein SM. Effect of interscalene brachial plexus block on the pulmonary function of obese patients: A prospective, observational cohort study. Anesthesia and Analgesia. 2017;**125**:313-319 PMID: 28609340. DOI: 10.1213/ANE.0000000000002180

[43] Desroches J. The infraclavicular brachial plexus block by the coracoid approach is clinically effective: An observational study of 150 patients. Canadian Journal of Anaesthesia. 2003;**50**:253-257 PMID: 12620948. DOI: 10.1007/BF03017794

[44] Rodriguez J, Taboada M, Valino C, Barcena M, Alvarez J. A comparison of stimulation patterns in axillary block: Part 2. Regional Anesthesia and Pain Medicine. 2006;**31**:202Y205

[45] Stein BE, Srikumaran U, Tan EW, Freehill MT, Wilckens JH. Lower-extremity peripheral nerve blocks in the perioperative pain management of orthopaedic patients: AAOS exhibit selection. The Journal of Bone and Joint Surgery. American Volume. 2012;**94**:e167 PMID: 23172334. DOI: 10.2106/JBJS.K.01706

[46] Paul JE, Arya A, Hurlburt L, Cheng J, Thabane L, Tidy A, et al. Femoral nerve block improves analgesia outcomes after total knee arthroplasty: A meta-analysis of randomized controlled trials. Anesthesiology. 2010;**113**:1144-1162 PMID: 20966667. DOI: 10.1097/ALN.0b013e3181f4b18

[47] Kwofie MK, Shastri UD, Gadsden JC, Sinha SK, Abrams JH, Xu D, et al. The effects of ultrasound-guided adductor canal block versus femoral nerve block on quadriceps strength and fall risk: A blinded, randomized trial of volunteers. Regional Anesthesia and Pain Medicine. 2013;**38**:321-325 PMID: 23788068. DOI: 10.1097/AAP.0b013e318295df80

[48] Jones MR, Novitch MB, Hall OM, Bourgeois AP, Jeha GM, Kaye RJ, et al. Fascia iliaca block, history, technique, and efficacy in clinical practice. Best Practice & Research. Clinical Anaesthesiology. 2019;**33**:407-413 PMID: 31791559. DOI: 10.1016/j.bpa.2019.07.011

[49] Candal-Couto JJ, McVie JL, Haslam N, Innes AR, Rushmer J. Pre-operative analgesia for patients with femoral neck fractures using a modified fascia iliaca block technique. Injury. 2005;**36**:505-510 PMID: 15755432. DOI: 10.1016/j.injury.2004.10.015

[50] Yun MJ, Kim YH, Han MK, Kim JH, Hwang JW, Do SH. Analgesia before a spinal block for femoral neck fracture: Fascia iliaca compartment block. Acta Anaesthesiologica Scandinavica. 2009;**53**:1282-1287 PMID: 19650803. DOI: 10.1111/j.1399-6576.2009.02052.x

[51] Kopp SL, Jacob AK, Hebl JR. Regional anesthesia in patients with preexisting neurologic disease. Regional Anesthesia and Pain Medicine. 2015;**40**:467-478 PMID: 26115188. DOI: 10.1097/AAP.0000000000000179

[52] Li D, Alqwbani M, Wang Q, Liao R, Yang J, Kang P. Efficacy of adductor canal block combined with additional analgesic methods for postoperative analgesia in total knee arthroplasty: A prospective, double-blind, randomized controlled study. The Journal of Arthroplasty. 2020;**35**:3554-3562 PMID: 32680754. DOI: 10.1016/j.arth.2020.06.060

[53] Soffin EM, YaDeau JT. Enhanced recovery after surgery for primary hip and knee arthroplasty: A review of the evidence. British Journal of Anaesthesia. 2016;**117**:iii62-iii72 PMID: 27940457. DOI: 10.1093/bja/aew362

[54] Kuang MJ, Ma JX, Fu L, He WW, Zhao J, Ma XL. Is adductor canal block better than femoral nerve block in primary total knee arthroplasty? The Journal of Arthroplasty. 2017;**32**:3238-3248.e3 PMID: 28606458. DOI: 10.1016/j.arth.2017.05.015

[55] Tran J, Giron Arango L, Peng P, Sinha SK, Agur A, Chan V. Evaluation

of the iPACK block injectate spread: A cadaveric study. Regional Anesthesia and Pain Medicine. 2019;**44**:689-694. DOI: 10.1136/rapm-2018-100355. PMID: 31061110.02

[56] Jinadu S, Pai P, Lai Y. Ambulatory knee replacements with IPACK block. Journal of Clinical Anesthesia. 2020;**60**:55-56 PMID: 31445181. DOI: 10.1016/j.jclinane.2019.08.021

[57] Sankineani SR, Reddy ARC, Eachempati KK, Jangale A, Gurava Reddy AV. Comparison of adductor canal block and IPACK block (interspace between the popliteal artery and the capsule of the posterior knee) with adductor canal block alone after total knee arthroplasty: A prospective control trial on pain and knee function in immediate postoperative period. European Journal of Orthopaedic Surgery and Traumatology. 2018;**28**:1391-1395 PMID: 29721648. DOI: 10.1007/s00590-018-2218-7

[58] Kim DH, Beathe JC, Lin Y, YaDeau JT, Maalouf DB, Goytizolo E, et al. Addition of infiltration between the popliteal artery and the capsule of the posterior knee and adductor canal block to periarticular injection enhances postoperative pain control in total knee arthroplasty: A randomized controlled trial. Anesthesia and Analgesia. 2019;**129**:526-535 PMID: 30234517. DOI: 10.1213/ANE.0000000000003794

[59] Vloka JD, Hadzić A, April E, Thys DM. The division of the sciatic nerve in the popliteal fossa: Anatomical implications for popliteal nerve blockade. Anesthesia and Analgesia. 2001;**92**:215-217 PMID: 11133630. DOI:10.1097/00000539-200101000-00041

[60] Prasad A, Perlas A, Ramlogan R, Brull R, Chan V. Ultrasound-guided popliteal block distal to sciatic nerve bifurcation shortens onset time: A prospective randomized double-blind study. Regional Anesthesia and Pain Medicine. 2010;**35**:267-271 PMID: 20921838. DOI: 10.1097/AAP.0b013e3181df2527

[61] Benzon HT, Jabri RS. Neuraxial anesthesia and peripheral nerve blocks in patietns on anticoagulants. In: Hadzic A, editor. NYSORA Textbook of Regional Anesthesia and Acute Pain Management. McGraw Hill; 2007. Available from: https://accessanesthesiology.mhmedical.com/content.aspx? bookid=413&sectionid=39828230

[62] Cashman JN. The mechanisms of action of NSAIDs in analgesia. Drugs. 1996;**52**(Suppl 5):13-23

[63] Al Farii H et al. The effect of NSAID son postfracture bone healing: A meta-analysis of randomized controlled trials. OTA International. 2021;**4**(2):e092

[64] Sampognaro G, Harrell R. Multimodal postoperative pain control after orthopaedic surgery. In: StatPearls [Internet]. Treasure Island, FL: StatPearls Publishing; 2021

[65] Scott L, Perry C. Tramadol—A review of its use in perioperative pain. Drugs. 2000;**60**(1):139-176

[66] Stiller C, Ludblad H, Weidnhielm L, Tullberg T, Grantinger B, Lafolie P, et al. The addition of tramadol to morphine via patient controlled analgesia does not lead to better postoperative pain relief after total knee artroplasty. Acta Anaesthesiologica Scandinavica. 2007;**51**:322-330

[67] Stubhaug A, Grimstad J, Breivik H. Lack of analgesic effect of 50 and 100 mg oral tramadol after orthopaedic surgery: A randomized, doublé-blind, placebo and standard active drug comparison. Pain. 1995;**62**:11-18

[68] Pang W-W, Mok MS, Lin C-H, Yang T-F, Huang M-H. Comparison of patient-controlled analgesia (PCA) with tramadol or morphine. Canadian Journal of Anesthesia. 1999;**46**:1030-1035

[69] Srivastava D, Hill S, Carty S, Rockett M, Bastable R, Knaggs R, et al. Surgery and Opioids: Evidence-based expert consensus guidelines on the perioperative use of opioids in the United Kingdom. British Journal of Anaesthesia. Jun 2021;**126**(6):1208-1216. DOI: 10.1016/j.bja.2021.02.030. Epub 2021 Apr 14. PMID: 33865553

[70] Sjövall S, Kokki M, Kokki H. Laparoscopic surgery: A narrative review of pharmacotherapy in pain management. Drugs. 2015;**75**:1867-1889

[71] Ordoñez Gallego A, González Barón M, Espinosa AE. Oxycodone: A pharmacological and clinical review. Clinical & Translational Oncology. 2007;**9**:298-307

[72] Don-won L, An J, Kim E, Lee J, Kim H. Comparison of oxycodone and fentanyl for postoperative patient-controlled analgesia after orthopedic surgery. Anesthesia and Pain Medicine. 2018;**13**:271-277

[73] Pergolizzi J, Magnusson P. Transdermal buprenorphine for acute pain in the clinical setting: A narrative review. Journal of Pain Research. 2021;**14**:871-879

[74] Desai SN, Badiger SV, Tokur SB, Naik PA. Safety and efficacy of transderal buprenorphine versus oral tramadol fo the treatment of post-operative pain following surgery for fracture neck of femur: A prospective, randomised clinical study. Indian Journal of Anaesthesia. 2017;**61**(3):225-229

[75] Xu X, Xie L, Liu H, Hu Y. Transdermal buprenorphine patch versus oral celecoxib for pain management after total knee arthroplasty: An open-label, randomized controlled trial. Orthopaedics & Traumatology: Surgery & Research. 2020;**106**(5):915-919

[76] Lopez MJ, Tadi P. Drug scheduling. Drug Enforcement Administration Drug Scheduling. [Updated 2022 Jun 23]. In: StatPearls [Internet]. Treasure Island (FL): StatPearls Publishing; Jan 2023. Available from: https://www.ncbi.nlm.nih.gov/books/NBK557426

[77] Pergolizzi J, Aloisi AM, Dahan A, et al. Current knowledge of buprenorphine and its unique pharmacological profile. Pain Practice. 2010;**10**(5):428-450

[78] Sittl R, Likar R, Nautrup BP. Equipotent doses of transdermal fentanil and transdermal buprenorphine in patients with cancer and nocancer pain: Results of a retropective cohort study. Clinical Therapeutics. 2005;**27**(2):225-237

Chapter 11

Postoperative Analgesia in Plastic Surgery Procedures

Daniela Arévalo-Villa, Andrea Figueroa Morales, Roberto de Jesús Jiménez-Contreras and Víctor M. Whizar-Lugo

Abstract

Advances in the knowledge of the secondary effects of acute postoperative pain have motivated anesthesiologists and surgeons to pay special attention to its prevention and correct management. Surgical procedures in plastic surgery are very varied and produce postoperative pain in direct relation to the site, type, and extent of surgery, with facial interventions being the least painful (with the exception of rhinoplasty) and the most painful being breast surgery, abdominoplasty, and extensive liposuctions due to the possibility of trauma to peripheral nerves and greater secondary inflammation. The combination of surgeries produces more intense post-surgical pain. There is insufficient data on the frequency and severity of pain after plastic surgery, be it reconstructive or cosmetic. Although opioids have been considered to be the cornerstone in the treatment of postsurgical pain, their use in plastic surgery patients must be carefully evaluated for various reasons that interfere with the results of this type of surgery. Similar to other surgical specialties, multimodal analgesia is now the most appropriate way to prevent and treat pain in these patients. This chapter is a comprehensive review of the management of acute postoperative pain in certain plastic surgery procedures, with emphasis on the multimodal approach.

Keywords: plastic, surgery, postoperative, pain, analgesia

1. Introduction

Postoperative pain (POP) is a subjective phenomenon, without a useful biological function, which varies with several factors such as the patient themselves, type of surgery, experience with previous surgeries, duration and extent of surgery, anesthetic technique, kind of perioperative care, individual characteristics and experiences, fear, and anxiety. The latest global survey from International Society for Aesthetic Plastic Surgery published in January 2023 reports a considerable increase in esthetic surgery worldwide, showing an overall 19.3% increase in procedures performed by plastic surgeons in 2021 with more than 12.8 million surgical procedures and 17.5 million non-surgical procedures performed globally. This equates to an increase of 33.3% over the last 4 years [1]. Paradoxically, the COVID-19 pandemic has increased plastic surgery procedures around the world; although the frequency of scheduled plastic surgery has apparently decreased in many countries, some procedures have increased as patients have free time for their cosmetic plans [2–5]. The top five most popular surgical procedures remain liposuction, breast augmentation, eyelid surgery, rhinoplasty, and abdominoplasty [1]. This notable increase in plastic surgeries has favored multiple advances not only in the surgical area, but in all anesthetic aspects, including the comprehensive management of POP. With increasing frequency, these types of surgeries are ambulatory or short stay, which tends to make the management of POP even more difficult, especially in the first post-surgical days.

Satisfactory POP management is mandatory for patient satisfaction. In patients undergoing thoracic and abdominal procedures, poor pain management has been related to pulmonary complications, cardiac ischemia, ileus, thromboembolism, and impaired immune function [6]. One of the greatest problems for adequate pain relief is due to inadequate physician familiarity with analgesic options available. Poorly controlled POP has been associated with deficient surgical outcomes, longer post-anesthesia care unit stays, poor pulmonary function, and higher readmission rates. The development of chronic pain after surgery, also called persistent postsurgical pain, is also related to uncontrolled acute POP and is recognized as a significant health problem [7]. On the one-day surgery basis, pain is one of the most prevalent problems, being as high as 58% 30 min after surgery in the undeveloped countries and up to 34.7% 48 h after discharge [6].

Up to date, multimodal analgesia is the most effective modality in the management of POP. This chapter reviews the importance of diagnosis, prevention, and timely management of POP in plastic surgery patients.

2. Postoperative pain in plastic surgery

Postoperative pain in patients undergoing plastic surgery procedures is a problem that has not been resolved and that implies serious management challenges. On one side, these patients are extremely demanding, with little or no tolerance for complications, especially POP. A growing number are tourist patients who have traveled many hours and sometimes thousands of kilometers by train, plane, or car only to be operated in remote places, where another language is often spoken, and customs as well as food are different from their original countries [8, 9]. Transgender and gender diversity patients are a steadily growing group requesting plastic surgery that requires meticulous care in a humanitarian sense, avoiding pejorative comments [10]. These factors produce stressful situations that make the proper management of POP even more difficult. An empathic patient-centered intervention can reduce preoperative anxiety and favor a faster surgical recovery, wound healing, and patient satisfaction.

On the other hand, some plastic surgeons and anesthesiologists do not have enough knowledge and sensitivity to address the timely treatment of POP [11, 12]. If we add the challenges of the current global crisis on the inappropriate and sometimes illegal use of opioids and other narcotics, the problem is even more difficult to address [13].

We did not find sufficient epidemiological data on the frequency and intensity of POP after plastic surgery, although it is known that the most painful procedures are breast surgery, abdominoplasty, extensive liposuction, and combined surgeries. In some studies, it is mentioned that plastic surgery, neurosurgery, orthopedics, and general surgery have the highest prevalence of severe POP varying from 10 to 75% [14–17].

3. Management of POP in plastic surgery

The POP approach should be started before surgery. This stage, known as pre-emptive analgesia, is based on preventing the development of spinal hyperexcitability and behaviors related to pain. The measures to prevent POP are basic and very simple in plastic surgery. During the initial evaluation, the anesthesiologist must gain the patient's trust by establishing a deep empathic relationship. The usual questioning and physical examination are not enough; the expectations of each patient must be known, and the reasons for their plastic surgery, and their personal and work environment are issues that facilitate this patient-anesthesiologist relationship. Pre-emptive analgesia includes the administration of an analgesic technique or drug with the aim of attenuating postoperative pain, hyperalgesia, and allodynia. In this phase, there is a wide range of possibilities, and several drugs must be used simultaneously. The preoperative combination of an NSAID, magnesium, ketamine, pregabalin, and an analgesic such as metamizole (dipyrone) or acetaminophen produces spectacular analgesic results [18–21].

3.1 Pharmacological management of POP in plastic surgery

The pharmacological management of POP in plastic surgery plays a fundamental aspect since it reduces complications, long stays, and costs, and favors rapid recovery after surgery. Various drugs and locoregional analgesia, including the tumescent technique widely used in plastic surgery, are part of multimodal analgesia programs in these patients [6, 22–24].

3.1.1 Opioids

Although opioids are the cornerstone in the treatment of POP, unfortunately plastic surgeons prescribe almost twice as many opioids as are required after outpatient surgeries, which continues to be a major factor in the globalized crisis of legal and illegal use of these drugs [12, 25–27]. Just to mention an example, in body-contouring surgeries, opioid overprescription is a proven routine among plastic surgeons. Bennett et al. [28] examined health insurance claims between 2001 and 2015 of patients with no history of opioid use who underwent body-contouring surgeries (abdominoplasty/panniculectomy, breast reduction, mastopexy, brachioplasty, and thigh plasty). They found that 6.1% of patients who had not previously received opioids developed persistent new use and 12.9% were exposed to high-risk prescriptions. Persistent opioid use was higher in high-risk prescription patients (9.2%), being the highest in thigh plasty (17.7%; 95% CI, from 0.03 to 0. 33). These researchers found high rates of mood disorders, anxiety, smoking, alcohol intake, neck pain, arthritis, and other pain disorders. In a study [29] of 56,773 patients undergoing body-contouring surgery, it was found that hydrocodone with paracetamol was the most prescribed opioid with an average of 17.9 days. These authors examined the comorbidities in this group of patients, finding that the cases with peripheral vascular disease and smoking were prescribed more opioids than patient without peripheral vascular disease (871.97 vs. 535.41; $p < 0.001$) and smoking (1069.57 vs. 440.84; $p < 0.001$). Those patients who developed surgical site infection, disruption of wound, and venous thromboembolism were prescribed a considerably greater dose of opioids (1213.63 vs. 561.59; $p < 0.001$). Another example of opioid overuse is augmentation mammoplasty where up to 91.2% of surgeons prescribe opioids, the most recommended being oxycodone with acetaminophen 47%, and hydrocodone with acetaminophen 38.3% [30].

Opioids primarily act on mu, kappa, and delta opioid receptor modulating the algesic response. Mu opiate receptor properties also include euphoria, sedation, anorexia, nausea, vomiting, respiratory depression as well as tolerance and opioid addiction. When prescribing opioids, it is important to consider patients' previous health conditions which could require chronic opioid use, or those conditions which may require higher doses in geriatric patients or patients with obstructive sleep apnea in which opioids may lead to airway obstruction.

Oliceridine is a new complex opioid, with potency similar to morphine, with no ceiling effect, which has fewer side effects than traditional opioids, although it can cause respiratory and CNS depression. It was approved by the US Food and Drug Administration in August 2020 for the intravenous treatment of moderate-to-severe acute pain in hospitalized patients. Although there is still not enough research on POP in plastic surgery, oliceridine could have a prominent place in these patients [31, 32].

3.1.2 Non-opioids

Acetaminophen (paracetamol) is one of the most frequently used analgesic agents. Despite the fact that it has been used for more than a century, its mechanism of action is not fully known, and is related to inhibition of CNS enzyme cyclooxygenase (COX) activities, with conflicting views on the COX isoenzyme/variant targeted by acetaminophen and on the nature of molecular interactions with these enzymes. It appears to selectively inhibit COX-2 by functioning as a reducing agent, although *in vitro* screening tests demonstrate low potency in inhibiting COX-1 and COX-2. In COX-1 transgenic mice, acetaminophen works through the inhibition of a variant of the COX-1 enzyme to mediate its analgesic and particularly thermoregulatory actions (antipyresis and hypothermia). Another possibility is that the descending inhibitory serotonergic pathway is potentiated to mediate the analgesic action of paracetamol, but without evidence of binding to serotonergic molecules. It has been proposed that AM404 (*N*-acylphenolamine), a paracetamol metabolite, activates the endocannabinoid1 and transient receptor potential vanilloid-1 (TRPV1) brain systems. Also, AM404 directly induces analgesia *via* TRPV1 receptors on terminals of C-fibers in the spinal dorsal horn [33, 34]. Consequently, acetaminophen induces analgesia by acting not only on the brain but also on the spinal cord.

It does not have the same gastric complications as other NSAIDs. A single dose of acetaminophen may reduce pain by 50%. However, its administration should be reduced in patients with liver malfunction, limiting its total dose to 2000 mg/day. In healthy patients, its total dose in 24 h should not be over 4000/day mg. Liver damage from acetaminophen is a rare secondary effect related to overdose.

3.1.3 Non-steroidal anti-inflammatory drugs (NSAIDs)

It is a group of non-opioid analgesics widely used in POP, although its potency is less than that of opioids and its side effects are extensive, especially with long-term use. Selective COX-2 inhibitors are linked to greater cardiovascular risk, while non-selective COX inhibitors are associated with higher gastrointestinal hazard. NSAIDs with lower renal excretion with phase 2 metabolism are less likely to induce adverse effects and drug-drug interactions [35].

NSAIDs, which act in COX-1 and COX-2, have demonstrated a suitable analgesic effect. However, many patients have restrictions on their administration due to the higher risk of bleeding. In 2021, a meta-analysis showed that in 151,031 surgical procedures, including esthetic surgeries, the NSAIDs were unlikely the cause of postoperative bleeding. Even though NSAIDs have little to no effect on bleeding, the difference in COX-1 and COX-2 is evident when we analyze platelet dysfunction. For nonselective COX-1, the platelet dysfunction was greater than with COX-2 inhibitors. According to Schoenbrunner et al., the best NSAID for plastic surgery has been meloxicam due to its one-day administration basis and the affinity to COX-2, which decreases its action in platelet function [6, 22]. COX-2 selective inhibitors are contraindicated in those with preexisting coronary artery disease because of their association with higher rates of cardiac events. COX-2 selective inhibitors and NSAIDs should also be avoided in patients with chronic or acute renal disease [26].

It has been shown that diclofenac associated with beta-lactam antibiotics could be useful in surgical infections caused by methicillin-resistant *Staphylococcus aureus* (MRSA) where implants are used [36], which would represent a considerable advance in augmentation mammoplasty with implants.

3.1.4 Other types of analgesics and adjuvants in POP

There is a group of drugs that are used as adjuvants in postoperative analgesia that have proven to be useful, although their advantages are still controversial [37–39]. Some of these drugs are reviewed below.

3.1.4.1 Gabapentinoids

These drugs are specific ligands for the $\alpha 2\delta$-1 subunit of voltage-gated calcium channels. Gabapentin, pregabalin, and mirogabalin have various pharmacological effects including antiepileptic, anti-anxiety, and analgesia, although this last effect is still controversial [40, 41]. A meta-analysis with 6201 patients found that the analgesic effect of both drugs is related to the doses used; pregabalin ($\geq$150 mg) was more effective than 75 mg, and gabapentin ($\geq$900 mg) if needed [38].

3.1.4.2 Ketamine

It is an extraordinary drug derived from phencyclidine. Synthesized in 1962 by Calvin Stevens at Parke Davis, it was first used in clinical anesthesia in 1965 by Corsen and Domino. It is a racemic mixture consisting of (S)- and (R)-ketamine, uncompetitive N-methyl-D-aspartate receptor antagonist. Although best characterized for its dissociative anesthetic properties, ketamine also has analgesic, anti-inflammatory, and antidepressant actions. It has been used as part of multimodal analgesia, from the pre-emptive phase, in the intraoperative period or in the immediate postoperative period. Sub-anesthetic doses of ketamine administered before induction or during trans-anesthesia have shown an analgesic effect in the postoperative period. It also has an important reduction in opioids and may reduce the hyperalgesia related to opioids [39]. Hallucinations are a disadvantage, although they are rare and can be prevented with a benzodiazepine administered as part of the preoperative medication.

3.1.4.3 Alpha-2 agonists

Alpha-2 adrenergic receptors are found in the central and peripheral nervous system, specifically in the pontine locus ceruleus, spinal cord tracts, rostral ventrolateral cord, and dorsal horn of the spinal cord. Clonidine, dexmedetomidine, and tizanidine are alpha-2 agonist drugs that modulate these centers, producing analgesia, sedation, bradycardia, and vasodilation without respiratory impairment. Its adjunctive effects to anesthesia are well known and are used as fundamental component of multimodal analgesia. In addition to their analgesic effect, they have been shown to reduce the use of perioperative opioids [18, 42–46].

3.1.4.4 Glucocorticoids

The use of glucocorticoids for postoperative pain is still controversial. They have a powerful anti-inflammatory effect through which their analgesic effect is hypothesized. Dexamethasone and methylprednisolone are the most used and can be administered perioperatively. They have also been used to reduce rebound pain that occurs with peripheral nerve blocks [47–49].

3.1.4.5 Metamizole (Dipyrone)

It is a non-opioid analgesic that has been demonized in some European countries and in the USA due to the possibility of death secondary to agranulocytosis, although it is one of the most used analgesics in the world since 1970. Its mechanism of action continues to be a question, having attributed to the inhibition of prostaglandin synthesis in peripheral tissues and in the central nervous system. Another recent theory mentions the modulation of CB1 and CB2 cannabinoid receptors [50, 51]. A randomized, double-blind, multiple-dose study in plastic surgery patients compared intramuscular metamizole 1 g (every 8 h) versus intramuscular diclofenac 75 mg (every 12 h), observing that dipyrone considerably decreased the requirement for meperidine as rescue analgesic in the first 18 h after surgery. This was also associated with significantly lower pain scores in patients receiving metamizole. Diclofenac had reduced side effects with thrombocytopenia and prolonged bleeding time in most patients [52].

At Lotus Med Group—a center specialized in plastic surgery—we use the analgesic management shown in **Table 1**, adjusting the doses according to the type of surgery, patient, analgesic response, and secondary effects. We believe that pre-emptive, intraoperative, and preventive multimodal analgesia is the best approach for the correct management of POP in plastic surgery. Of course, the analgesic approach must always consider an empathetic and pleasant environment for each patient, offering continuous follow-up in the immediate and mediate postoperative period. Using this analgesic approach, we have not had cases of persistent postoperative pain.

3.1.4.6 Local anesthetics

Local anesthetics (LA) inhibit neuronal action potentials *via* voltage-gated sodium channel blockade. LA for postoperative analgesia is a safe option as long as the total doses administered are monitored to avoid dangerous side effects, including death. These drugs can be administered by injection into the wound, subcutaneously, by tumescent infiltration, intravenously, by the neuroaxial route, in peripheral nerve

Pre-surgery	Intraoperative	First 24–48 h	Analgesics at home**
Etoricoxib 90 mg oral	Fentanyl 50 up to 250 μg	Nalbuphine 5–10 mg i.v. /6 h	Tramadol 25–300 mg/day Codeine 15–60 mg/day Oxycodone 5–15 mg/6 h Acetaminofen 500 mg/4–6 h Etoricoxib 90–120 mg/day Celecoxib 100–400 mg/day Ibuprofen 200–400 mg/6–8 h Diclofenac 25, 50 or 100 mg/6 h Pregabaline 75 mg/12 h
Clonidine 0.1 mg oral	Morphine 10–30 mg	Metamizole 2 gr iv drip/12 h	
Melatonine 10 mg oral	Nalbuphine up to 30 mg	Ketorolac 30 i.v./8 h	
Magnesium sulfate 2 g i.v.	Clonidine 75–250 μg*	Pregabaline 75 mg/12 h. oral	
Metamizole 1 gr i.v.			
Dexamethasone 8 mg i.v.			

**Added to bupivacaine during spinal anesthesia.*
***Combination of 1 opioid, 1 NSAID or acetaminofen, plus pregabaline.*

Table 1.
Perioperative analgesia plan for adult patients in plastic surgery.

blocks, interpleural, or in transdermal patches. Local infiltration of LA is a simple technique widely used by plastic surgeons; from the various tumescent solutions where local anesthetics are mixed—primarily lidocaine—to some regional blocks. LA toxicity is a controversial issue among anesthesiologists and plastic surgeons. The maximum safe doses of tumescent lidocaine have been reported to be 28 mg/kg without liposuction and 45 mg/kg with liposuction, doses that produce serum lidocaine concentrations below toxic levels [53]. The American Society of Plastic Surgeons Practice Advisory on Liposuction recommends not to exceed a maximum dose of 35 mg/kg and only as part of a wetting solution [54]. Intravenous perioperative lidocaine decreases the incidence and intensity of chronic postoperative pain: initial bolus dose of 1.5 mg/kg followed by a continuous lidocaine infusion of 1.5 mg/kg during surgery.

3.2 Regional analgesia

The role of regional anesthesia to treat POP in plastic surgery procedures has been widely discussed [22–24, 55, 56]. Some authors suggest that this method of analgesia may reduce the incidence of pain by many mechanisms. Blocking the nerves interferes the transmission of nociceptive input from peripheral nerves, giving as result the reduced inflammation of the nerves and the activation of glial cells. This technique also reduces the opioid consumption during and after surgery, decreases PONV, and cuts lengths of stay as well as costs. Regional blocks as well as neuroaxial analgesia are extensively used in many specialties and have become a component of many Enhanced Recovery After Surgery (ERAS) protocols. Epidural analgesia has demonstrated to improve pain management at 1 year after surgery, and recent studies have shown that peripheral nerve blocks have the same analgesic outcomes [57].

3.2.1 Peripheral nerve blocks

The increasingly frequent use of ultrasound-guided peripheral blocks favors the anesthetic and analgesic effects, decreasing side effects and complications, improves

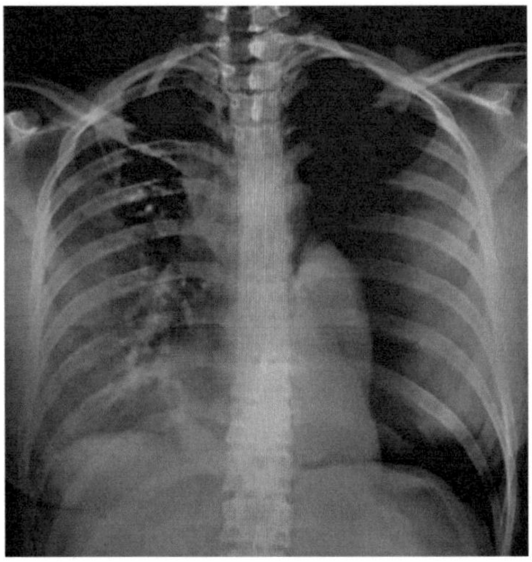

Figure 1.
Left pneumothorax secondary to intraoperative intercostal block for POP in breast implants.

comfort and quality of recovery of the patient, and decreases chronic post-surgical pain and dependence on opioid drugs. In plastic surgery, the most used for mammary surgery are PEC I and II, erector spinae plane block, and thoracic paravertebral blocks, and some surgeons like to perform proximal intercostal nerve blockade.

Although some studies have mentioned the possibility that PECS blockade combined with multimodal analgesia does not reduce intraoperative and/or PACU opioid consumption in women undergoing ambulatory breast surgery [58], the meta-analysis by Grape et al. [59] including 1026 patients in 16 trials concludes that there is moderate-to-high-level evidence that PECS blocks provide postoperative analgesia after breast surgery when compared with no regional technique. Ahiskalioglu et al. [60] evaluated the use of bilateral ultrasound-guided serratus plane block in 40 patients undergoing breast reduction, concluding that it is a safe technique in the treatment of POP, in addition to reducing the consumption of opioids.

Intercostal blocks are easy to perform, although they have some complications such as rapid absorption of LAs and, of course, the possibility of pneumothorax, as shown in **Figure 1**.

For abdominoplasty, the transversus abdominis plane (TAP) block, rectus abdominis muscle block, and erector spinae plane block [60–62], as well as analgesia by tumescent infiltration using lidocaine, ropivacaine, or levobupivacaine [63, 64], produce excellent relief of POP.

4. Conclusions

The prevention and treatment of POP are mandatory in the comprehensive management of patients undergoing plastic surgery—be it cosmetic or reconstructive—since moderate-to-intense post-surgical pain generates negative physiological changes that affect rapid recovery, prolong hospitalization, higher readmission rates, high costs, and interference with patient satisfaction. Multimodal analgesia has proven to be the best regimen in the comprehensive management of these patients, requiring an approach that includes medications combined with non-pharmacological techniques.

Although opioids have been the cornerstone in the treatment of pain secondary to surgery, the indiscriminate use of opioids for POP should be avoided.

Proper management of POP is an important determinant in the rapid recovery of patients and the return to their daily activities.

Conflict of interest

The authors declare no conflict of interest.

Author details

Daniela Arévalo-Villa[1*], Andrea Figueroa Morales[1],
Roberto de Jesús Jiménez-Contreras[1] and Víctor M. Whizar-Lugo[2]

1 Department of Anesthesia, Centro Médico ABC, México City, Mexico

2 Department of Anesthesia, Lotus Med Group, Tijuana, Mexico

*Address all correspondence to: d.arevalovilla@gmail.com

References

[1] Global Survey 2021. Full report and press releases [Internet]. Isaps. org. [cited 2023 Sep 28]. Available from: https://www.isaps.org/discover/about-isaps/globalstatistics/reports-and-pressreleases/globalsurvey-2021-full-reportand-press-releases/

[2] Mortada H, Alawaji ZH, Aldihan RA, Alkuwaiz LA, Alshaalan SF, et al. Impact of the Coronavirus Disease 2019 pandemic on the patterns and characteristics of plastic surgery practice: A retrospective comparative study of before and during the pandemic. Cureus. 2022;**14**(9):e29722. DOI: 10.7759/cureus.29722

[3] Moss WD, Pires GR, Samlowski E, Webb J, DeAngelo MM, et al. Characterizing the volume of surgery and post-operative complications during the COVID-19 pandemic. Langenbeck's Archives of Surgery. 2022;**407**(8):3727-3733. DOI: 10.1007/s00423-022-02605-6

[4] Qiao Z, Deng Y, Wang X, Sun Y, Xiong X, et al. The impact of COVID-19 on plastic and reconstructive surgery in China: A single-centre retrospective study. Journal of Plastic, Reconstructive & Aesthetic Surgery. 2023;**76**:160-168. DOI: 10.1016/j.bjps.2022.10.033

[5] Che K, Wang K, Yuan Y, Zhang Z, Li F, Li Q. Trend of academic productivity in plastic surgery and the impact of COVID-19: A bibliometric analysis. The Journal of Craniofacial Surgery. 2023;**34**(2):454-460. DOI: 10.1097/SCS.0000000000009021

[6] Schoenbrunner AR, Joshi GP, Janis JE. Multimodal analgesia in the aesthetic plastic surgery: Concepts and strategies. Plastic and Reconstructive Surgery. Global Open. 2022;**10**(5):e4310. DOI: 10.1097/GOX.0000000000004310

[7] Richebé P, Capdevila X, Rivat C. Persistent postsurgical pain: Pathophysiology and preventative pharmacologic considerations. Anesthesiology. 2018;**129**(3):590-607. DOI: 10.1097/ALN.0000000000002238

[8] Whizar-Lugo V, Flores-Carrillo JC, Campos-León J, Parra-Beltrán P, Azamar-Llamas D. Perioperative care of tourist-patients. Journal of Anesthesia and Critical Care: Open Access. 2015;**3**(6):00119. DOI: 10.15406/jaccoa.2015.03.00119

[9] May DM. Ambulatory anesthesia for cosmetic surgery in Brazil. Current Opinion in Anaesthesiology. 2016;**29**(4):493-498. DOI: 10.1097/ACO.0000000000000361

[10] Lai A, Johnson R. World professional association for transgender health guidelines: 2022 surgical treatment updates in the standards of care for transgender and gender diverse people. Neurourology and Urodynamics. 2022;**42**(5):900-902. DOI: 10.1002/nau.25099

[11] Torabi R, Bourn L, Mundinger GS, Saeg F, Patterson C, et al. American Society of Plastic Surgeons member post-operative opioid prescribing patterns. Plastic and Reconstructive Surgery. Global Open. 2019;**7**(3):e2125. DOI: 10.1097/GOX.0000000000002125

[12] Oberhofer HM, Rao A, Carlson JT, Mast BA, Simmons CJ, et al. Opioid prescribing practices among plastic surgeons: Results of the 2019 American Society of Plastic Surgeons opioid survey. Annals of Plastic Surgery.

2022;**88**(6):665-673. DOI: 10.1097/SAP.0000000000003145

[13] Wang AMQ, Retrouvey H, Wanzel KR. Addressing the opioid epidemic: A review of the role of plastic surgery. Plastic and Reconstructive Surgery. 2018;**141**(5):1295-1301. DOI: 10.1097/PRS.0000000000004332

[14] Cabedo N, Valero R, Alcón A, Gomar C. Prevalence and characterization of postoperative pain in the postanaesthesia care unit. Revista Española de Anestesiología y Reanimación. 2017;**64**(7):375-383. DOI: 10.1016/j.redar.2016.11.006

[15] Domínguez HG, Sandoval LCG, Domínguez CLG. Prevalencia de dolor postquirúrgico. Acta Médica Grupo Ángeles. 2016;**14**(2):84-89

[16] Gramke HF, de Rijke JM, van Kleef M, Raps F, Kessels AG, et al. The prevalence of postoperative pain in a cross-sectional group of patients after day-case surgery in a university hospital. The Clinical Journal of Pain. 2007;**23**(6):543-548. DOI: 10.1097/AJP.0b013e318074c970

[17] Chung F, Ritchie E, Su J. Postoperative pain in ambulatory surgery. Anesthesia and Analgesia. 1997;**85**(4):808-816. DOI: 10.1097/00000539-199710000-00017

[18] Nair A, Rangaiah M, Borkar N. Efficacy and safety of oral tizanidine premedication as pre-emptive analgesia in adult patients undergoing elective surgeries—A systematic review. Saudi Journal of Anaesthesia. 2023;**17**(2):214-222. DOI: 10.4103/sja.sja_780_22

[19] Klifto KM, Elhelali A, Payne RM, Cooney CM, Manahan MA, Rosson GD. Perioperative systemic nonsteroidal anti-inflammatory drugs (NSAIDs) in women undergoing breast surgery. Cochrane Database of Systematic Reviews. 2021;**11**(11):CD013290. DOI: 10.1002/14651858.CD013290.pub2

[20] Dahl JB, Møiniche S. Pre-emptive analgesia. British Medical Bulletin. 2004;**71**:13-27. DOI: 10.1093/bmb/ldh030

[21] Whizar LV, Cisneros CR, Reyes AMA, Campos LJ. Anestesia para cirugía facial cosmética. Anest Mex. 2005;**17**:117-131

[22] Schoenbrunner AR, Janis JE. Pain management in plastic surgery. Clinics in Plastic Surgery. 2020;**47**(2):191-201. DOI: 10.1016/j.cps.2019.12.001

[23] Mahaalit-Aribawa GN, Wiryana M, Agung-Senapathi T, Parami P. Pain management in plastic surgery. In: Whizar-Lugo VM, editor. Anesthesia Topics for Plastic and Reconstructive Surgery. London, UK: Intechopen; 2018. pp. 102-128. DOI: 10.5772/intechopen.79302. Chapter 6

[24] Saffari TM, Saffari S, Brower KI, Janis JE. Management of acute surgical pain in plastic and reconstructive surgery. Plastic and Reconstructive Surgery [Internet]. 2023. Publish Ahead of Print. DOI: 10.1097/prs.0000000000010694

[25] Rose KR, Christie BM, Block LM, Rao VK, Michelotti BF. Opioid prescribing and consumption patterns following outpatient plastic surgery procedures. Plastic and Reconstructive Surgery. 2019;**143**(3):929-938. DOI: 10.1097/PRS.0000000000005351

[26] Barker JC, Joshi GP, Janis JE. Basics and best practices of multimodal pain management for the plastic surgeon. Plastic and Reconstructive Surgery. Global Open. 2020;**8**(5):e2833. DOI: 10.1097/GOX.0000000000002833

[27] Martínez CF, Hernández CE. ¿Sabes que es realmente el fentanilo? Anest Mex. 2023;**35**(2):345-349

[28] Bennett KG, Kelley BP, Vick AD, Lee JS, Gunaseelan V, et al. Persistent opioid use and high-risk prescribing in body contouring patients. Plastic and Reconstructive Surgery. 2019;**143**(1):87-96. DOI: 10.1097/PRS.0000000000005084

[29] Mundra L, Garossi K, Iorio M, Mathes D, Winocour J, Kaoutzanis C. Opioid-prescribing patterns in body contouring surgery. Aesthetic Surgery Journal [Internet]. 2023;**43**(9):978-985. DOI: 10.1093/asj/sjad117

[30] Crystal DT, Cuccolo NG, Plewinski MJ, Ibrahim AMS, Sinkin JC, et al. Assessment of opioid-prescribing practices in breast augmentation: Future directions for prescribing guidelines. Annals of Plastic Surgery. 2021;**86**(1):11-18. DOI: 10.1097/SAP.0000000000002430

[31] Singla NK, Skobieranda F, Soergel DG, Salamea M, Burt DA, et al. APOLLO-2: A randomized, placebo and active-controlled phase III study investigating oliceridine (TRV130), a G protein-biased ligand at the μ-opioid receptor, for management of moderate to severe acute pain following abdominoplasty. Pain Practice. 2019;**19**(7):715-731. DOI: 10.1111/papr.12801

[32] Simpson KN, Fossler MJ, Wase L, Demitrack MA. Cost–effectiveness and cost-benefit analysis of oliceridine in the treatment of acute pain. Journal of Comparative Effectiveness Research. 2021;**10**(15):1107-1119

[33] Ayoub SS. Paracetamol (acetaminophen): A familiar drug with an unexplained mechanism of action. Temperature (Austin). 2021;**8**(4):351-371. DOI: 10.1080/23328940.2021.1886392

[34] Mallet C, Desmeules J, Pegahi R, Eschalier A. An updated review on the metabolite (AM404)-mediated central mechanism of action of paracetamol (acetaminophen): Experimental evidence and potential clinical impact. Journal of Pain Research. 2023;**16**:1081-1094. DOI: 10.2147/JPR.S393809

[35] Ribeiro H, Rodrigues I, Napoleão L, Lira L, Marques D, et al. Non-steroidal anti-inflammatory drugs (NSAIDs), pain and aging: Adjusting prescription to patient features. Biomedicine & Pharmacotherapy. 2022;**150**:112958. DOI: 10.1016/j.biopha.2022.112958

[36] Zhang S, Qu X, Tang H, Wang Y, Yang H, et al. Diclofenac resensitizes methicillin-resistant Staphylococcus aureus to β-lactams and prevents implant infections. Advanced Science. 2021;**8**(13):2100681. DOI: 10.1002/advs.202100681

[37] Low YH, Gan TJ. NMDA receptor antagonists, gabapentinoids, α-2 agonists, and dexamethasone and other non-opioid adjuvants: Do they have a role in plastic surgery? Plastic and Reconstructive Surgery. 2014;**134**(4 Suppl. 2):69S-82S. DOI: 10.1097/PRS.0000000000000703

[38] Hu J, Huang D, Li M, Wu C, Zhang J. Effects of a single dose of preoperative pregabalin and gabapentin for acute postoperative pain: A network meta-analysis of randomized controlled trials. Journal of Pain Research. 2018;**11**:2633-2643. DOI: 10.2147/JPR.S170810

[39] O'Neill RC, Hayes KD, Davison SP. Safety of postoperative opioid alternatives in plastic

surgery: A systematic review. Plastic and Reconstructive Surgery. 2019;**144**(4):991-999. DOI: 10.1097/PRS.0000000000006074

[40] Verret M, Lauzier F, Zarychanski R, Perron C, Savard X, et al. Perioperative use of gabapentinoids for the management of postoperative acute pain: A systematic review and meta-analysis. Anesthesiology. 2020;**133**(2):265-279. DOI: 10.1097/ALN.0000000000003428

[41] Dauri M, Faria S, Gatti A, Celidonio L, Carpenedo R, et al. Gabapentin and pregabalin for the acute post-operative pain management. A systematic-narrative review of the recent clinical evidences. Current Drug Targets. 2009;**10**(8):716-733. DOI: 10.2174/138945009788982513

[42] Whizar LV, Gómez-Ramírez IA, Cisneros-Corral R, Martínez-Gallegos N. Intravenous dexmedetomidine vs. intravenous clonidine to prolong bupivacaine spinal anaesthesia. A double blind study. Anest Mex. 2007;**19**:143-146

[43] Whizar-Lugo V, Flores-Carrillo J, Preciado-Ramírez S. Intrathecal clonidine as spinal anaesthesia adjuvant - is there a magical dose? In: Topics in Spinal Anaesthesia. London, UK, Croatia: Intechopen; 2014. pp. 97-121. DOI: 10.5772/58712. Chapter 5

[44] Kaye AD, Chernobylsky DJ, Thakur P, Siddaiah H, Kaye RJ. Dexmedetomidine in enhanced recovery after surgery (ERAS) protocols for postoperative pain. Current Pain and Headache Reports. 2020;**24**(5):21. DOI: 10.1007/s11916-020-00853-z

[45] Chen R, Sun S, Li Y, Dou X, Dai M, et al. Efficacy and safety evaluation of dexmedetomidine for postoperative patient controlled intravenous analgesia: A systematic review and meta-analysis. Frontiers in Pharmacology. 2022;**13**:1028704. DOI: 10.3389/fphar.2022.1028704

[46] Fernández Martin MT, Alvarez Lopez S, Aldecoa A-SC. Role of adjuvants in regional anesthesia: A systematic review. Revista Española de Anestesiología y Reanimación. 2023;**70**(2):97-107. DOI: 10.1016/j.redare.2021.06.006

[47] Jensen KK, Brøndum TL, Leerhøy B, Belhage B, Hensler M, et al. Preoperative, single, high-dose glucocorticoid administration in abdominal wall reconstruction: A randomized, double-blinded clinical trial. Surgery. 2020;**167**(4):757-764. DOI: 10.1016/j.surg.2019.12.007

[48] Jensen KK, Brøndum TL, Belhage B, Hensler M, Arnesen RB, et al. Preoperative steroid in abdominal wall reconstruction: Protocol for a randomised trial. Danish Medical Journal. 2016;**63**(8):A5260

[49] Gao M, Li Y, Yu J, Li W, Qin S, et al. The effects of intravenous dexamethasone on rebound pain after nerve block in patients with ankle fracture: A randomized controlled trial. Journal of Pain Research. 2023;**16**: 1127-1136. DOI: 10.2147/JPR.S399660

[50] de Oliveira DR, Maia RC, de Carvalho França PR, Fernandes PD, Barbosa G, et al. 2-arylpropionic acid pyrazolamides as cannabinoid CB2 receptor inverse agonists endowed with anti-inflammatory properties. Pharmaceuticals (Basel). 2022;**15**(12):1519. DOI: 10.3390/ph15121519

[51] Stessel B, Lambrechts M, Evers S, Vanderstappen C, Callebaut I,

et al. Non-opioid analgesics and the endocannabinoid system. Balkan Medical Journal. 2020;**37**(6):309-315. DOI: 10.4274/balkanmedj.galenos.2020.2020.6.66

[52] Saray A, Büyükkocak U, Cinel I, Tellioglu AT, Oral U. Diclofenac and metamizol in postoperative analgesia in plastic surgery. Acta Chirurgiae Plasticae. 2001;**43**(3):71-76

[53] Klein JA, Jeske DR. Estimated maximal safe dosages of tumescent lidocaine. Anesthesia and Analgesia. 2016;**122**(5):1350-1359. DOI: 10.1213/ANE.0000000000001119

[54] Iverson RE, Lynch DJ. American Society of Plastic Surgeons Committee on Patient Safety. Practice advisory on liposuction. Plastic and Reconstructive Surgery. 2004;**113**(5):1478-1490; discussion 1491-5. DOI: 10.1097/01.prs.0000111591.62685.f8

[55] Bagatin D, Bagatin T, Šakić K, Deutsch J, Nemrava J, Šimičević D. Optimal analgesia for breast surgery enhanced recovery in day surgery. Acta Clinica Croatica. 2022;**61** (Suppl. 2):49-56. DOI: 10.20471/acc.2022.61.s2.06

[56] ElHawary H, Joshi GP, Janis JE. Practical review of abdominal and breast regional analgesia for plastic surgeons: Evidence and techniques. Plastic and Reconstructive Surgery. Global Open. 2020;**8**(12):e3224. DOI: 10.1097/GOX.0000000000003224

[57] Homsy C, Lindsey JT. Regional anesthetic blocks in plastic surgery using portable ultrasound: A simplified approach. Annals of Plastic Surgery. 2019;**82**(6S Suppl. 5):S374-S379. DOI: 10.1097/SAP.0000000000001805

[58] Uribe AA, Weaver TE, Echeverria-Villalobos M, Periel L, Pasek J, et al. Efficacy of PECS block in addition to multimodal analgesia for postoperative pain management in patients undergoing outpatient elective breast surgery: A retrospective study. Frontiers in Medicine (Lausanne). 2022;**9**:975080. DOI: 10.3389/fmed.2022.975080

[59] Grape S, Jaunin E, El-Boghdadly K, Chan V, Albrecht E. Analgesic efficacy of PECS and serratus plane blocks after breast surgery: A systematic review, meta-analysis and trial sequential analysis. Journal of Clinical Anesthesia. 2020;**63**:109744. DOI: 10.1016/j.jclinane.2020.109744

[60] Ahiskalioglu A, Yayik AM, Demir U, Ahiskalioglu EO, Celik EC, Ekinci M, et al. Preemptive analgesic efficacy of the ultrasound-guided bilateral superficial serratus plane block on postoperative pain in breast reduction surgery: A prospective randomized controlled study. Aesthetic Plastic Surgery. 2020;**44**(1):37-44. DOI: 10.1007/s00266-019-01542-y

[61] Williams L, Iteld L. Moving toward opioid-free breast surgery: Regional blocks and a novel technique. Clinics in Plastic Surgery. 2021;**48**(1):123-130. DOI: 10.1016/j.cps.2020.09.003

[62] Liheng L, Siyuan C, Zhen C, Changxue W. Erector spinae plane block versus transversus abdominis plane block for postoperative analgesia in abdominal surgery: A systematic review and meta-analysis. Journal of Investigative Surgery. 2022;**35**(9):1711-1722. DOI: 10.1080/08941939.2022.2098426

[63] Bagatin D, Bagatin T, Nemrava J, Ivelj MŠ, Deutsch J, Šakić K. Influence

of local infiltration analgesia on postoperative pain in abdominoplasty patients. Acta Clinica Croatica. 2019;**58**(Suppl. 1):23-28. DOI: 10.20471/acc.2019.58.s1.03

[64] Šakić K, Bagatin D, Bagatin T, Šakić L, Jeleč V, et al. Comparison of different surgical procedures with local infiltration analgesia in day surgery. Acta Clinica Croatica. 2019;**58**(Suppl. 1):67-73. DOI: 10.20471/acc.2019.58.s1.10

Chapter 12

Chronic Postoperative Pain

Saúl Gilberto Almeida-Návar, Nexaí Reyes-Sampieri, Jose Trinidad Morelos-Garcia, Jorge Mario Antolinez-Motta and Gabriel Ivan Herrejón-Galaviz

Abstract

Understanding the definition of pain has imposed numerous challenges toward pain practitioners. The pain experience phenomena are complicated to understand, and this construct goes beyond biomedical approaches. Persistent pain as a disease implicates changes that include modified sensory feedback within the somatosensory system. It has been documented that different anatomical restructuring in nociceptive integration and adaptations in nociceptive primary afferents and perception conduits are present in persistent pain situations. Chronic postoperative pain (CPOP) is known as a particular disorder, not only associated with a specific nerve damage or manifestation of a unique inflammatory response but also with a mixture of both. The occurrence of CPOP varies substantially among the literature and depends on the kind of procedure. There are reports informing that 10 to 50% of the patients undergoing common procedures had CPOP, and 2 to 10% of patients complained of severe pain. Systematic review has been performed trying to identify the Holy Grail, none showed sufficient evidence to guide CPOP treatment, and multimodal approaches must be tried in large randomized controlled trials (RCTs) to provide robust evidence as evidence-based management for CPOP still lacking.

Keywords: chronic, pain, postsurgical, persistent, postoperative

1. Introduction

It is necessary to fully understand the latest definition of pain, and it is well implied that this subject has imposed several challenges toward pain practitioners, requiring some adjustments over the years. The revised International Association for the Study of Pain recommended that the concept of pain should be revised to "An unpleasant sensory and emotional experience associated with, or resembling that associated with, actual or potential tissue damage." It is well known that this definition has suffered changes over the years because of the complexity of this experience where it can differ broadly in intensity, quality, and duration and has varied pathophysiology mechanisms and implications [1–4].

Pain as an aporia. The approach toward the treatment of pain needs to be multidisciplinary, that is why all the patients with persistent pain invite a clinical judgment of psychosocial susceptibility. The pain experience phenomena are very complex to understand; in these recent years, we still practice a linear (biomedical) approach where we do not find success in terms of treatment; this construct goes beyond biomedical approaches. We as doctors need to accept that there are various cases where the solution is beyond our expertise and very difficult to comprehend. That is why currently the concept of pain constitutes an aporia (paradox), but as pain physicians we have the ethical obligation to engage this disease to benefit the patient that is experiencing pain [3–5].

Persistent pain as a disease implicates changes that include modified sensory feedback within the somatosensory system. It has been documented that different anatomical restructuring in nociceptive integration and adaptations in nociceptive primary afferents and perception conduits are present in persistent pain situations. This pain state involves a biopsychosocial model where the biological aspect is not always the answer; it is well described that pain states defined as "functional" are expressed, and there is no evidence that justifies this pathology, only psychological and environmental causes. There are other complex cases known as nociplastic pain; in this situation, there is no clear evidence of tissue harm causing the triggering of peripheral nociceptors or sign for disease or alteration of the somatosensory system responsible of the pain state [3, 4].

The proposition made by these authors regarding this construct brings up to mind the concept of biopsychosocial framework, where we can talk about the body-mind dualism proposed by Rene Descartes. It is very difficult to define pain, we as doctors try always to rule out potential biological causes that provoke pain, forgetting that sometimes there is a biopsychosocial framework responsible of this incident [2, 3].

Anesthesiologists play an important role in preventing this pathology, and they have all the tools and knowledge necessary to avoid this type of pain. Chronic postoperative pain (CPOP) is known as a particular disorder that not only associated with a specific nerve damage or manifestation of a unique inflammatory response but also associated with a mixture of both [3].

2. Incidence

The occurrence of CPOP varies substantially among the literature and depends on the kind of procedure. It has been documented 20–50% for mastectomy, around 50–80% for amputation, and 5–65% for thoracotomy. There are reports informing that 10 to 50% of the patients undergoing common procedures had CPOP, and 2 to 10% of patients complained of severe pain [3].

In 2015, there was a study implemented in 21 European hospitals, and the significant outcomes were a 6-month postsurgical extension. There were reports of modest severe CPOP in 24% of patients and exceedingly severe CPOP in 16% of patients. At the end of a 12-month follow-up, the incidence of CPOP was reduced 12 to 24% depending on the duration and the intensity of pain in the first 24 hours. With this information they concluded that the pain duration in the first 24 hours is considered as a risk factor for the progress of CPOP [3].

CPOP is a well-defined pathology that affects patients who were exposed to a certain type of surgery (affection of 5 to 75% of surgical patients). This type of pain is very important to consider because it affects importantly the quality of life and results in patient disability and mandate additional health and social expenses. When the evidence points out that the cause of the pain is neuropathic the condition exacerbates, with an occurrence of CPOP fluctuating from 6 to 68% of the cases, differing on distinct surgery scenarios. The first publication that identified prior surgery as a cause of chronic pain came from a pain clinic in Northern England in 1998 where Chrombie et al. found that almost one in four patients attributed their pain to an operation. Since that time, it has been shown that depending on the type of surgery, the incidence of CPOP is anywhere between 5 and 85%. The frequency over the last years has not changed over time, the exact mechanisms of CPOP remain uncertain, and the treatment continues to be a challenge [3, 6, 7].

3. Criteria for diagnosis

The criteria for CPOP suggested by Macrae and Davies in 1999 are as follows:

1. The pain must have established following surgery.

2. The pain is of at least 2 months in length.

3. Other sources of pain have been eliminated.

4. The likelihood that the pain in continuing from a preexisting problem must be investigated and exclusion attempted.

The recently suggested criteria are as follows:

1. The pain progresses after a surgical event or rises in intensity after the surgical process.

2. The pain is of at least 3–6 months duration and significantly affects quality of life.

3. The pain is a perpetuation of acute postsurgery pain or progresses after an asymptomatic stage.

4. The pain is contained to the surgical field, projected to the innervation zone of a nerve located in the surgical field, or referred to a dermatome.

5. Other causes of the pain should be eliminated [3, 6, 8].

4. Risk factors

Some circumstances allow the establishment of CPOP, an important risk factor in the type of surgery, although there are some other factors to be included in these perpetuation of conditions such as acute severe postsurgical pain, biopsychosocial affection, demographics, and lack of control on the intensity of pain in the near postoperative stage. Actual data informs us about the gross number of surgeries made annually throughout the world. This gives us an idea of the estimate for the general frequency of 10% for CPOP, meaning that around 23 million patients per year are suffering with this painful situation [3].

4.1 Abdominal surgery

In 2014, a report integrated liver donation patients that had a frequency of CPOP of 31% in 6th month and 27% in 12th month and concluded that several risk factors were involved, detecting female gender, young patients, and psychological distress associated with pain states as potential elements for the development of CPOP. In 2015, a retrospective study documented a CPOP frequency of 17% following colorectal surgery and concluded that potential risk for CPOP were redo surgery for anastomotic leakage, inflammatory bowel disease, and acute severe pain. Similarly, in 2016, an analysis found that women who encountered an abdominally based autologous breast reconstruction surgery found a frequency of CPOP of 23–24% in a 6–12 month follow-up; they concluded that the leading cause for the development of CPOP at 6 months is poor control of severe acute pain in the first 24-0 hour post-surgery [3].

4.2 Breast surgery

Modern analysis has determined a frequency of CPOP of 30–60% with an existence of moderate to severe pain of 14%. It is well documented that preoperative distress may be considered as a key element for CPOP progression, and another nonsignificant risk factors are <65 years of age, breast reconstructive intervention, axillary lymphadenectomy, bad control of acute severe pain in the postsurgical period, inferior presurgical diastolic blood pressure, and signs of somatosensorial damage associated with pain at 1 week [3].

4.3 Cardiac surgery

Actual reports in patients after sternotomy document a frequency of CPOP at 3 months to be 43%, diminishing substantially over time reporting 11% at 12 months and 3.8% at 5 years. In 2016, several authors concluded that a positive neuropathic sign like hyperalgesia around the sternotomy wound on day 4 of surgery was not linked with CPOP at month 4th and 6th. However, they concluded that the biopsychosocial sphere, age, gender, obesity, complex surgeries, history of previous procedures, osteoarthritis, and poor management of acute severe pain in the postsurgical period may be linked with and increased risk for development of CPOP [3].

4.4 Hysterectomy

A couple of studies discovered a global frequency of CPOP of 26% at 6 months after laparoscopic or vaginal hysterectomy and a rate of moderate-to-severe CPOP of 10.2 and 9.0%, correspondingly, at 3 and 12 months after these surgical approaches. In a report developed in 2015, they found that procedures performed with this methodology had a strong relationship with CPOP if they had a story of tobacco usage, acute severe pain in the first hours of the postsurgical period, history of infection related to the procedure, and anxiety associated with the surgery [3].

4.5 Inguinal hernia surgery

A study conducted in 2015 associated with inguinal hernia surgery after 1 year of the surgical procedure reported a frequency of CPOP of 43% in patients aged

18–40 years old, 29% in the 40–60 age interval, and barely 19% for patients with 60 years and above. In patients where the inguinal repair was made with mesh, there is a strong link with CPOP development with a frequency of 9.3% at 3 months and intensity of CPOP was related with robust hemodynamic preoperative changes [3].

4.6 Total knee arthroplasty

The latest data on osteoarthritis patients document a CPOP frequency of 58%. At 2014, an analysis discovered a strong relationship with severe pain intensity throughout a knee active flexion an extension exercise preceding a total knee arthroplasty (TKA) with moderate to severe pain at 6 months. A meta-analysis conducted by Lewis et al. followed patients during 3 months to 7 years undergoing TKA; they discovered that there was a strong linkage with CPOP and alterations in the biopsychosocial sphere, presurgical knee pain, other chronic pain states associated with current pathology, and catastrophizing [3].

4.7 Thoracic surgery

Actual reports related to this type of approaches document a frequency of 57% for CPOP at 3 months, 39–56% at 6 months, and 50% at 1 year. Regarding other thoracic approaches that are minimally invasive like the ones that are video-assisted have a lower frequency of CPOP that extend 11–30% [3].

4.8 Thyroidectomy

Evidence on a report of 2016 sustains a frequency of 37% for CPOP at 3 months preceding minimally invasive video-assisted thyroidectomy. Different studies document a frequency of neuropathic pain preceding thyroidectomy of 12–9% at 3rd and 6th month, respectively. There is a strong linkage with presurgical anxiety and doubt respecting the procedure with the development of CPOP [3].

5. Key definitions

Acute pain is considered as a particular state where the patient experiences a biopsychosocial reaction to tissue lesion related to inflammatory states, and it can experience discomfort and the management can be very complex. Generally acute pain is limited to a time interval but, in some cases, it may perpetuate and transform in chronic pain. One of the purposes of acute pain is human preservation, and it limits conducts that place the patient in danger and promotes tissue healing [5].

Chronic pain is characterized as pain that endures beyond tissue healing and the related metabolic and inflammatory disruption in the body. This kind of pain affects completely the biopsychosocial sphere and promotes patient disability and hospital costs in an important manner [6].

Persistent postsurgical pain is documented in 10–50% of patients that undergo surgery; depending on the magnitude of the surgery some of these patients will experience acute severe pain, if this initial situation perpetuates patients can develop chronic pain. It is well documented that one of the main factors for persistent postsurgical pain is poor control of acute pain in the first hours of the postsurgical event. The IASP's classification system for chronic pain syndromes makes a particular description as "a persistent pain state that endures two or more months of the surgical event that cannot be explained by other causes." This is accompanied by different changes that affect the somatosensorial system that lead to central and peripheral sensibilization that finally will manifest as chronic pain and worsen the patient's quality of life [6].

6. Factors related to the development of CPOP

There are different causes that perpetuate CPOP, and there is an argument that places an important relationship of acute severe pain associated with nerve injury as a crucial element of this continuum and subsequently the presence of neuropathic pain. The surgeries that are related with CPOP in this circumstance (nerve injury) are breast reconstruction, thoracotomy, and amputation. It is important to mention that there is not always evidence of nerve damage in patients with CPOP, and those who have nerve damage will not develop CPOP constantly. There is evidence that one of the principal elements of CPOP progression is repeated and intense triggering of primary afferents which encourages peripheral and central sensitization [3, 6, 7].

If the outcome of the surgery is nerve injury the patient will experience inflammatory changes that will encourage electrical discharges and early ectopic events in the nociceptive pathways. There may be observed adjacent propagation of intact nociceptive afferents nearby areas innervated by injured afferents, and this added to changes induced by damage progression in the somatosensorial system developed by this continuum of events posterior to perioperative pain incitement [2, 5]. CPOP progression is defined by neuroplastic changes resulting from neurotrophic factors and the interface neuron-microglia, and in association with the outcomes of inhibitory modulation. If this particular situation is not managed, CPOP can progress and manifest different alterations that can develop a complex pain syndrome that perpetuates over time and the treatment may impose an important challenge [3, 6, 7].

6.1 Chronicity of acute pain

This event leads to variations in the peripheral and central somatosensory system associated with inflammatory and biochemical modifications that in combination aggravate this pain syndrome. It has been described several changes in distinct receptors where we can punctuate the erratic activation of N-methyl-D-aspartate (NMDA) receptors that leads to liberation of glutamate in the spinal cord at the dorsal horn originated by peripheral afferents, and additionally ectopic and erratic triggering of nerves injured during the surgical event. These neuroplastic changes lead to peripheral and central sensitization resulting in an exaggerated response to pain [3, 6, 9].

Positive symptoms of neuropathic pain include allodynia and hyperalgesia that strongly suggest signs of central sensitization, and these states frequently express incongruence concerning the intensity and perception of the painful stimulus. Hyperalgesia is usually seen throughout the tissue recovery course; if this event persists and it is allowed to progress, it may be related to CPOP progression. Without a doubt, the degree and length of central and peripheral sensitization and the mechanisms causing disparity among the descendent and ascending pain nociceptive pathways; these circumstances fluctuate enormously during the progress of acute severe pain and CPOP [3, 6, 9].

6.2 Animal experiment basic research

In the 90s of the last century, a specific animal model was designed to recognize mechanisms that are essential for lesion-induced postsurgical pain. A plantar lesion model was described to study particular evidence of the fundamental neurophysiology of lesion-induced pain. Somehow this model describes that many of the mechanisms responsible of pain as inflammation, antigen-induced or neuropathic pain are not responsible for incisional pain and vice versa. A couple of concepts are revealed during an induced lesion, primary hyperalgesia that develops at the side of the incision and subsequently in an area adjacent to the injury when it comes to secondary hyperalgesia after various days once the lesion has established [3, 6, 9].

6.3 Spinal sensitization after surgical incision

It has been documented that several elements that are used to avert central sensitization and CPOP progression in other pain models were unsuccessfully after surgical incision. The initial reports regarding this model identified that NMDA receptor antagonists were futile in the context of CPOP prevention. Somehow this information guided to the hypothesis that the surgical lesion originates another type of spinal sensitization compared to other pain entities. This type of sensitization is perpetuated after this model (plantar incision) is sustained by the afferent limit of sensitized nociceptors on the non-NMDA/AMPA receptor group, which in conjunction are accountable for no evoked pain and hyperalgesia after surgical lesion. There are several substances responsible of mechanical/heat hyperalgesia that act on the ascending and descending nociceptive pathways, and the stimulation of GABAA and GABAB receptors somehow diminish this response, but there is no evidence on attenuation of no evoked pain by this specific reaction [3, 6, 9].

6.4 Peripheral sensitization after incision

In the initial stages of surgical lesion, the reports on plantar incision provide substantial evidence of peripheral C and A delta fiber sensitization in the acute phase. There is analysis in behavior and neurophysiological experiments where muscle nociceptors play a crucial function in the cause of no evoked protecting conduct after surgical lesion. Although a skin surgical lesion without involvement of muscle tissue lesion seems to be accountable for promoting mechanical hyperalgesia posterior to surgical lesion. This confirms that a muscle injury is not required for the appearance of positive signs of neuropathic pain on the patient [3, 6, 9].

6.5 Neuroplastic changes in the brain after incision

Actual evidence confirms that presurgical or postsurgical exposure to distressing elements like immobilization and force swimming test does not make difference on pain awareness to incitements, such as mechanical, hot, and cold, and it somehow delays the period of lesion provoked hyperalgesia after surgical incision. There are reports linked to abolishing stress-induced hyperalgesia by the withdrawal of adrenal gland and impeding the activation of glucocorticoid receptors [3, 6, 9].

7. Prevention of chronic postoperative pain

As already mentioned, CPOP has a deleterious effect on the quality of life of the person who suffers from it, causing important economic, social and family repercussions. The risk factors that predispose to the presentation of this entity have already been enumerated, and how it can be added to each other for its presentation. That is why efforts should focus on correcting modifiable causes, such as the characteristics of the surgery, anesthesia techniques, and the use of pharmacological prophylaxis [10].

Although it is not a certainty that CPOP can be avoided, diverse reports have determined that the frequency is lower when risk factors are identified [2]. Preoperative factors, such as localized pain far from the surgical site, chronic use of opioids, and mood disorders such as anxiety and depression, will alert about the patients who need multimodal strategies such as regional anesthesia, hyperalgesic drugs, etc. [11]. The objective will then be to reduce the mechanisms of central and peripheral sensitization [12]. Regional anesthesia, peripheral nerve blocks, and intravenous infusions of various anesthetic adjuvants have been shown to be beneficial in the prevention and reduction of chronic postoperative pain [12].

Among the most accepted and recommended drugs are NSAIDs, as long as there is not contraindication, and in conjunction with a protective medication for the gastric mucosa, or a selective COX2 (cyclooxygenase-2) inhibitor (maximum 7 days, and do not use in cases with increased risk of a thrombotic event) [11].

Intravenous infusions of local anesthetics such as lidocaine have recently shown good results in the prevention and control of immediate postoperative pain, which it means into a lower prevalence of persistent pain after recovery. Some study protocols talk about loading doses followed by infusions of around 1–2 mg/kg/h with encouraging results [11]. There is no evidence indicating that gabapentinoids reduce or prevent CPOP, so they are not recommended [11, 13, 14]. Although no prophylactic role has been found in the use of gabapentinoids, they have been used successfully in the long-term treatment of persistent postoperative neuropathic chronic pain [15, 16].

The use of ketamine has been justified by its properties at the NMDA receptor level and its antagonism in the dorsal horn of the spinal cord. In combination with other agents, it has been shown to be effective and safe [16].

The mechanism of local anesthetics in chronic postoperative pain perhaps due to the decrease of neuronal inflammation and glial activation, avoiding chemical, structural, and functional changes [15].

The use of opioids alone for the postoperative period has not been associated with reductions in the incidence of postoperative pain; to the contrary it produces opioid-induced hyperalgesia and prolonged use after surgery. The use of opioids in multimodal therapy with NSAIDs is recommended to reduce the effects of acute inflammation induced by cyclooxygenases and the sensitization of peripheral nerve fibers [17].

Regional anesthesia and nerve blocks are perhaps one of the most useful measures for the prevention and management of CPOP. It is recommended that, when it is identified a patient with risk factors for developing CPOP, regional anesthesia can be prioritized whenever possible or, otherwise, general anesthesia using local anesthetics such as lidocaine, alpha agonists (dexmedetomidine), inhibitors of NMDA receptors (ketamine), and plexus or peripheral nerve block techniques, to maximize the analgesic effect during the intraoperative period and during the acute phase of post-surgical recovery.

In abdominal surgeries, for example, improvement in acute postoperative pain and a lower incidence of CPOP have been found with the use of a transverse abdominal plane block plus placement of a continuous perfusion catheter [8]. Neck procedures under general anesthesia and a bilateral superficial cervical plexus block have been described with good results and lower levels of acute postoperative pain. This strengthens the idea that maintaining pain control during the first 24 hours after surgery reduces the risk of pain chronicity. In spinal surgery, erector spinae blockade techniques have been described for postoperative pain control with good long-term results [5].

Prevention strategies must be applied in those patients considered to be at high risk, perform a complete preoperative evaluation before and after the procedure, and develop preventive strategies establishing an appropriate therapeutic plan for each particular patient.

8. Diagnosis of chronic postsurgical pain

It has currently been considered that it is mandatory to identify the risk factors and the possibilities to prevent CPOP, because it has been studied by different authors as a preventable sequel and some others classify it as iatrogenic, since the triggering mechanisms are already known. The diagnosis of this syndrome is already described in the International Statistical Classification of Diseases (ICD-11) of 2019 [18]. One of the most common and devastating forms of presentation is postsurgical chronic neuropathic pain, both for intensity levels as well as functional alterations for the patient.

The medical history is an essential part of the patient evaluation. The characteristics of the pain, intensity, triggering and mitigating agents, as well as the history of pain prior and after the surgical procedure, in addition to the functionality report, will be important indicators that will guide us in the diagnosis. The use of scales to assess the pain, visual analog scale, or numerical analog scale can be a useful guide in the follow-up of the cases. Patients with limited pain communication, such as patients with cognitive impairment or who have a condition that makes it impossible for them to speak, should not be overlooked. For this, behavioral tools such as Pain in Advanced Dementia (PAINAD), Behavioral Pain Scale, have been created for evaluation of these type of patients [18]. Another aspect that should not be forgotten is obtaining a description of persistent postoperative pain with the degree of functional impairment and the extent of disability in the patient [19]. In the study of Stamer in 2019, the associated variables with persistent postoperative pain 6 months after surgery were found: young patients, with intense pain before the surgical procedure or severe pain in the 24 hours following postoperative recovery. In the gender relationship, men showed a risk 3.6 times greater than women; the most commonly associated surgeries were orthopedic, abdominal, and thoracic related to breast cancer [16, 18, 19].

Diagnostic criteria for this entity have not yet been described; however, the recent definition of the IASP can guide evaluation and timely treatment [10]. The type of surgery also helps to establish diagnostic suspicion, for example, in breast cancer CPOP presents 65% of the time as neuropathic pain, mainly as intercostal neuralgia and post-mastectomy pain syndrome, followed by musculoskeletal pain. Another aspect that should not be forgotten when obtaining a description of persistent postoperative pain is the degree of functional impairment and the extent of disability in the patient [19].

9. Chronic postoperative pain management

As we mentioned in previous lines, CPOP may be ominous as patient experience more emotional distress and tends to have higher pain intensity compared to those with an insidious onset, making it even more difficult to manage; biopsychosocial approach is recommended to understand and treat the source properly; rehabilitation programs must be included [10].

Exhaustive clinical examination focusing on identifying sensory dysfunction areas due to nerve damage, previous medical history detailing prior pain medications, impact on quality of life and limitation for daily-basis activity should be considered as first step to chronic pain treatment to identify the mechanisms by which chronic pain is being produced or was produced in the first place; during assessment before any intervention, possible postsurgical complication must be ruled out, complications due to surgical technic or preoperative patient's conditions such as malignancy recurrence or intestinal anastomosis leak are extremely frequent [20]. Once knowing the mechanisms and its etiology, a treatment line can be established based on its causes. Prevention is the cornerstone to avoid the perpetuation of pain; however, in case of CPOP, multimodal treatment would be the ideal choice [21].

One of the main techniques in the management is regional anesthesia, whether applied neuraxially or as peripheral nerve blocks. It has an effect through the modulation of pain to avoid central and peripheral sensitization; this technique has the ability to transform moderate or severe pain to mild, and the purpose is to avoid central sensitization or reduce the probability of it on the long run. Regional anesthesia techniques vary according to each surgical procedure, or the site of pain that the patients specify [22, 23].

Other pharmacological alternatives are gabapentinoids, through the inhibition of the alpha(2) delta unit regulate neuronal excitation, preventing the over excitation and sensitization. However, the adverse effects are significant (dizziness, nausea, vision changes), and relatively high doses are usually required for control or therapeutic efficacy [24]. Alpha2 agonists belong to another group of drugs used to relieve, reduce, and prevent pain, and these effects are produced through an agonist effect on alpha receptors in the spinal cord, causing analgesia and an opioid-sparing consumption produced by synergistic effect, the representative drugs are dexmedetomidine and clonidine, but both have important adverse effects such as sedation. Thus, there are no presentations for alpha2 agonists in the outpatient setup, and they can only be used in the hospital environment under strict surveillance. More scientific evidence is required to investigate the efficacy/safety of this therapy, since there are few important clinical studies that support these effects [25]. COX 2 inhibitors and paracetamol are adjuvants that could be used to reduce and control pain, both are involved in the regulation of the inflammatory response mediated by pro-inflammatory cytokines, by inhibiting the synthesis of prostaglandins, acute-phase reactants whose inhibition could prevent or avoid the risk of perpetuating central and peripheral pain sensitization. Currently, there are no randomized clinical studies which use COX 2 inhibitors and acetaminophen for the treatment of CPOP, though both drugs belong to treatment strategies in a multimodal analgesia scheme [26].

10. Conclusions

Above all, opioids and the use of regional anesthesia are probably the first-line treatment strategies for CPOP as they can provide an almost immediate and significant benefit in the setting of acute severe pain. Within opioids, mild-acting ones such as tramadol as well powerful opioids (oxycodone, buprenorphine, fentanyl) which have numerous presentations and routes of administration for pain control are part of the tool setting of the anesthesiologist in the acute pain scenario. However adverse effects such as sedation, nausea, constipation, and opiophobia limit its uses; it is indispensable for the anesthesiologists in the acute pain scenario to have a robust knowledge of the opioid pharmacokinetics and pharmacodynamics for adequate outcomes, as well a proper training in regional anesthesia and ultrasound management to provide an effective execution of this techniques [27].

Systematic review has been performed trying to identify the Holy Grail, all the interventions included were unimodal, none showed sufficient evidence to guide CPOP treatment, multimodal approaches must be tried in large randomized controlled trials (RCTs) to provide robust evidence as evidence-based management for CPOP still lacking.

Author details

Saúl Gilberto Almeida-Návar[1*], Nexaí Reyes-Sampieri[1],
Jose Trinidad Morelos-Garcia[2], Jorge Mario Antolinez-Motta[3]
and Gabriel Ivan Herrejón-Galaviz[4]

1 Instituto Nacional de Ciencias Médicas y Nutrición Salvador Zubirán, Ciudad de México, México

2 Hospital del Prado, Tijuana, Mexico

3 Hospital General Dr. Manuel Gea González, Ciudad de México, México

4 Spine and Pain Baja, Mexicali, Mexico

*Address all correspondence to: drsalmeida89@gmail.com

References

[1] Aydede M. Does the IASP definition of pain need updating? Pain Reports. 2019;**4**(5):e777. DOI: 10.1097/PR9.0000000000000777

[2] Cohen M, Quintner J, van Rysewyk S. Reconsidering the international association for the study of pain definition of pain. Pain Reports. [Internet]. 2018;**3**(2):e634. DOI: 10.1097/pr9.0000000000000634

[3] Lopes A, Seligman Menezes M, Moreira A, de Barros G. Chronic postoperative pain: Ubiquitous and scarcely appraised: Narrative review. Brazilian Journal of Anesthesiology. 2021;**71**(6):649-655. DOI: 10.1016/j.bjane.2020.10.014

[4] Quintner JL, Cohen ML, Buchanan D, Katz JD, Williamson OD. Pain medicine and its models: Helping or hindering? Pain Medicine. 2008;**9**(7):824-834. DOI: 10.1111/j.1526-4637.2007.00391.x

[5] Raja SN, Carr DB, Cohen M, Finnerup NB, Flor H, Gibson S, et al. The revised international association for the study of pain definition of pain: Concepts, challenges, and compromises: Concepts, challenges, and compromises. Pain. 2020;**161**(9):1976-1982. DOI: 10.1097/j.pain.0000000000001939

[6] Chapman CR, Vierck CJ. The transition of acute postoperative pain to chronic pain: An integrative overview of research on mechanisms. The Journal of Pain. [Internet]. 2017;**18**(4):359.e1-359.e38. DOI: 10.1016/j.jpain.2016.11.004

[7] Correll D. Chronic postoperative pain: Recent findings in understanding and management. F1000Res [Internet]. 2017;**6**:1054. DOI: 10.12688/f1000research.11101.1

[8] Schug SA, Lavand'homme P, Barke A, Korwisi B, Rief W, Treede R-D, et al. The IASP classification of chronic pain for ICD-11: Chronic postsurgical or posttraumatic pain: Chronic postsurgical or posttraumatic pain. Pain [Internet]. 2019;**160**(1):45-52. DOI: 10.1097/j.pain.0000000000001413

[9] Pogatzki-Zahn EM, Segelcke D, Schug SA. Postoperative pain—From mechanisms to treatment. Pain Reports [Internet]. 2017;**2**(2):e588. DOI: 10.1097/pr9.0000000000000588

[10] Chen Y-YK, Boden KA, Schreiber KL. The role of regional anaesthesia and multimodal analgesia in the prevention of chronic postoperative pain: A narrative review. Anaesthesia. 2021;**76**:8-17. DOI: 10.1111/anae.15256

[11] Aubrun F et al. Revision of expert panel's guidelines on postoperative pain management. Anaesthesia Critical Care & Pain Medicine. 2019;**38**(4):405-411. DOI: 10.1016/j.accpm.2019.02.011

[12] Gan TJ. Poorly controlled postoperative pain: Prevalence, consequences, and prevention. Journal of Pain Research. 2017;**10**:2287-2298. DOI: 10.2147/JPR.S144066

[13] Martinez V, Pichard X, Fletcher D. Perioperative pregabalin administration does not prevent chronic postoperative pain: Systematic review with a meta-analysis of randomized trials. Pain. 2017;**158**(5):775-783. DOI: 10.1097/j.pain.0000000000000838

[14] Clark JD. Chronic postoperative pain: Preventable or inevitable? Anesthesiology. 2021;**135**(2):215-217. DOI: 10.1097/ALN.0000000000003839

[15] Gulur P, Nelli A. Persistent postoperative pain: Mechanisms and modulators. Current opinion in Anaesthesiology. [Internet]. 2019;**32**(5):668-673. DOI: 10.1097/aco.0000000000000770

[16] Anwar S et al. Prolonged perioperative use of pregabalin and ketamine to prevent persistent pain after cardiac surgery. Anesthesiology. 2019;**131**(1):119-131. DOI: 10.1097/ALN.0000000000002751

[17] Feller L, Khammissa RAG, Bouckaert M, Ballyram R, Jadwat Y, Lemmer J. Pain: Persistent postsurgery and bone cancer-related pain. The Journal of International Medical Research [Internet]. 2019;**47**(2):528-543. DOI: 10.1177/0300060518818296

[18] Stamer U, Ehrler M, Lehmann T, Meissner W, Fletcher D. Pain-related functional interference in patients with chronic neuropathic postsurgical pain: An analysis of registry data. Pain. 2019;**160**(8):1856-1865. DOI: 10.1097/j.pain.0000000000001560

[19] Haroutiunian S, Nikolajsen L, Finnerup NB, Jensen TS. The neuropathic component in persistent postsurgical pain: A systematic literature review. Pain. [Internet]. 2013;**154**(1):95-102. DOI: 10.1016/j.pain.2012.09.010

[20] Steyaert A, Lavand'homme P. Prevention and treatment of chronic postsurgical pain: A narrative review. Drugs [Internet]. 2018;**78**(3):339-354. DOI: 10.1007/s40265-018-0866-x

[21] Althaus A, Arránz Becker O, Moser K-H, Lux EA, Weber F, Neugebauer E, et al. Postoperative pain trajectories and pain chronification-an empirical typology of pain patients. Pain Medicine [Internet]. 2018;**19**(12):2536-45. DOI: 10.1093/pm/pny099

[22] Fujii T, Shibata Y, Akane A, Aoki W, Sekiguchi A, Takahashi K, et al. A randomised controlled trial of pectoral nerve-2 (PECS 2) block vs. serratus plane block for chronic pain after mastectomy. Anaesthesia [Internet]. 2019;**74**(12):1558-1562. DOI: 10.1111/anae.14856

[23] Woolf CJ. Central sensitization: Implications for the diagnosis and treatment of pain. Pain [Internet]. 2011;**152**(3 Suppl):S2-S15. DOI: 10.1016/j.pain.2010.09.030

[24] Verret M, Lauzier F, Zarychanski R, Perron C, Savard X, Pinard A-M, et al. Perioperative use of gabapentinoids for the management of postoperative acute pain: A systematic review and meta-analysis. Anesthesiology [Internet]. 2020;**133**(2):265-279. DOI: 10.1097/ALN.0000000000003428

[25] Jain G, Bansal P, Ahmad B, Singh DK, Yadav G. Effect of the perioperative infusion of dexmedetomidine on chronic pain after breast surgery. Indian Journal of Palliative Care [Internet]. 2012;**18**(1):45-51. DOI: 10.4103/0973-1075.97354

[26] Richebé P, Capdevila X, Rivat C. Persistent postsurgical pain: Pathophysiology and preventative pharmacologic considerations. Anesthesiology [Internet]. 2018;**129**(3):590-607. DOI: 10.1097/ALN.0000000000002238

[27] Dahl JB, Kehlet H. Postoperative Pain and its Management. Elsevier, Churchill Livingstone; 2006:635-651

Chapter 13

Physical Analgesia: Methods, Mechanisms and Algorithms for Post-Operative Pain

Ivet B. Koleva, Borislav R. Yoshinov, Teodora A. Asenova and Radoslav R. Yoshinov

Abstract

Physical analgesia is the application of physical modalities for pain relief. Our objective is to present the potential of some physical factors and correspondent methods of application; and to explain their mechanisms of action. For pain reduction we use: low and middle frequency electric currents (e.g. TENS, interferential currents), electrostatic field (Deep oscillation), magnetic field, light (including Laser), some mineral waters and peloids, physiotherapy (e.g. analytic exercises, mechanotherapy, post-isometric relaxation, massage), reflexotherapy (e.g. acupuncture, acupressure). In rehabilitation practice, we use reflectory connections between the surface of the body and the internal organs (cutaneous-visceral, subcutaneous-visceral, proprio-visceral, periostal-visceral). The theory of Melzack and Wall for gate-control explains some effects of physical factors. We propose our own theory for explanation of mechanisms of physical analgesia. We propose our concept about rehabilitation algorithms in diseases of the nervous and locomotor systems, accentuating on conditions after surgical intervention (neurosurgical and orthopedic operations, including joint endoprosthesis and limb amputations). We present some of our own results in patients with post-operative pain.

Keywords: pain, physical factors, analgesia, electric currents, magnetic field, photo-therapy, physiotherapy

1. Introduction

According the International Association for the Study of Pain (IASP) pain is an unpleasant sensory and emotional experience associated with actual or potential tissue damage, or described in term of such damage [1]. Pain is provoked by stimulation of nociceptors (pain receptors), by modifications in sensory roads, or in cerebral zones. Pain perception depends on different physical, chemical or psychological factors [2].

The biological importance of pain is the safeguard of the organism from negative stimuli (external or internal), liberating a defensive reaction. The French philosopher Rene Descartes [3] explains the shielding character of pain and its capacity to unchain a reaction as a self-protective reflex.

In 1959, Willem Noordenbos [4] expressed the hypothesis for the multi-synaptic transmission of pain-signal.

In 1965, the British physiologist Patrick Wall and the Canadian psychologist Ronald Melzack published the article "Pain Mechanisms: A New Theory" [5]. According the theory of gate control, in the spinal medulla exists a controlling mechanism, which is closed in response to the normal stimulation of fast fibers of tactile sense, but is open if the slow fibers of pain perception transport numerous and intensive sensory signals. A subsequent stimulation of the fast fibers can close the gate and interrupt these signals [6, 7].

Pain perception has different levels: receptors, sensory roots, posterior columns of the spinal medulla, thalamus opticus, reticular formation, and cerebral cortex. Actually, we apply three groups of theories for explanation of pain perception: specific, non-specific and combined [8–10]. Specific theories accept the existence of specific pain receptors—nociceptors. According non-specific theories: pain perception depends on decoding (at spinal level) of temporo-spatial organization of patterns—signals, perceived by intensive stimulation of non-specific receptors. The third group of theories accept both theories.

The pathogenesis of pain determines the differentiation of *acute and chronic (persistent) pain; nociceptive and neuropathic pain.* In clinical practice, every pain has elements of nociceptive and neuropathic elements, and this fact is the base of our *therapeutic impotence* behind pain [8, 9].

In rehabilitation practice, we observe different types of pain: *Nociceptive* and *Neuropathic* pain, *Central* pain, *Post-operative pain* (in neurological and neurosurgical conditions); *Degenerative and Inflammatory pain* (in rheumatologic diseases); *Traumatic (Post-traumatic) pain; Post-operative pain; Fibromyalgia or Myofascial pain, pain due to muscle dysbalance; Tendinopathy pain* or *Ligamentar pain* (in orthopedic and traumatic conditions); *Cancer pain (oncological); Phantom pain* [2, 10].

The Declaration of Montréal of the International Pain Summit of the International Association for the Study of Pain (IASP) categorizes chronic pain as a serious health problem and proclaims access to pain management as a fundamental human right [11].

2. Physical analgesia: methods

Pain management is very important for the successful rehabilitation. Different members of our multi-disciplinary multi-professional rehabilitation team are included in the pain treatment. The role of the medical doctors—specialists in Physical and Rehabilitation Medicine is crucial in this process [12, 13].

Physical analgesia is the application of physical factors for pain management. The anti-pain effect of physical modalities is significant [2, 10, 14]. Physical analgesia has not side effects and can be combined with other therapies [15].

In physical analgesia, we apply several physical modalities (**Table 1**).

- *Preformed modalities*: Electric currents; Magnetic fields; Ultra-sound; Light beams: infra-red, ultra-violet or Laser [2, 10, 14, 16–25];

- *Natural modalities*: Kryo-factors; Thermo-agents; Mineral waters; Hydro and balneo-physiotherapy techniques; Peloids; Physiotherapy techniques—analytic exercises or soft-tissue techniques [2, 10, 15, 25–33];

Types of physical modalities	Methods	Procedures
Preformed modalities	*Electrotherapy*	Low frequency currents (galvanic, diadynamic currents); Low frequency modulated middle frequency currents (sinusoidal-modulated, interferential, Kots currents); Trans-cutaneous electroneurostimulation (TENS)
		High frequency currents (diathermy, ultra-high frequency currents, decimeter and centimeter waves)
		Deep Oscillation
	Magnetotherapy	Low frequency pulsed magnetic field
		Ultra-sound and phonophoresis with NSAIDs;
	Phototherapy	infra-red, ultra-violet, visible light; LASER (laser-therapy)
Natural modalities	*Cryo-therapy*	ice, cold packs, cold compresses
	Thermo-therapy	hot packs, hot compresses
	Hydro- and Balneo-therapy	douches, baths, piscine
	Hydro and balneo-physiotherapy	underwater massage, under water exercises,
	Peloidotherapy	fango therapy, thermal mud, sea lye compresses
	Physiotherapy	Analytic exercises; stretching, post-isometric relaxation
	Manual therapy	Traction (distraction), mobilization, manipulation
	Massage	Manual massage or with devices; periostal, connective tissue massage, etc.
Reflectory methods	*Reflexotherapy*	Electrotherapy, thermotherapy and physiotherapy in reflectory points and zones
		Acupuncture and Acupressure
		Laserpuncture and Laseracupuncture
Telerehabilitation techniques		

Table 1.
Methods of Physical analgesia.

- *Reflectory methods*: electrotherapy, thermotherapy and physiotherapy in reflectory points and zones; acupuncture, laserpuncture, acupressure, etc [34].

- *Telerehabilitation techniques* [35, 36].

3. Physical analgesia: mechanisms

The gate-control theory [5] is widely applied in physical medicine, especially for explanation of physical analgesia, using the principle of the "contra-stimulation"—final effect reticence by stimulation of inhibiting systems, or else final effect stimulation by embarrassment of inhibiting systems [37, 38]. Investigations of J. Gacheva demonstrated that the selective electrostimulation of tactile Aβ-nerve fibers (with high velocity of conduction) provokes a previous stimulation of suppressive neurons, they inhibit the tardily arrived nociceptive stimuli of A-δ and C-fibers (with slower conduction velocity) [37].

At peripheral level, the direct anti-adaptive electrostimulation of receptors probably provokes a hyperpolarization with a decrease of the sensibility of the nociceptors.

A direct low frequency electrical stimulation of the Aδ and C fibers may cause an analgesic effect.

During last years, the development of the physical medicine proved the existence of some reflectory connections in the human body, based on the theory for the metameric structure of the embryo during intra-uterine development. In physical analgesia, we apply the following **groups of reflectory connections** (**Figure 1**).

- *cutaneous-visceral*—between skin and internal organs (e.g. zones of Head, used in iontophoresis),
- *between the subcutaneous connective tissue and visceras* (e.g. zones of Leube–Dicke, applied in connective massage),
- *proprio-visceral* and *motor-visceral*—between proprio-receptors and internal organs (e.g. zones of Mackenzie, used in the physiotherapeutic method of Mackenzie),
- *periostal-visceral*—between periostium and internal organs (e.g. zones of Vogler–Krauss, used in periosteal massage).

We consider that physical modalities may provoke an analgesic effect by different pathogenetic mechanisms (**Figure 2**, **Table 2**).

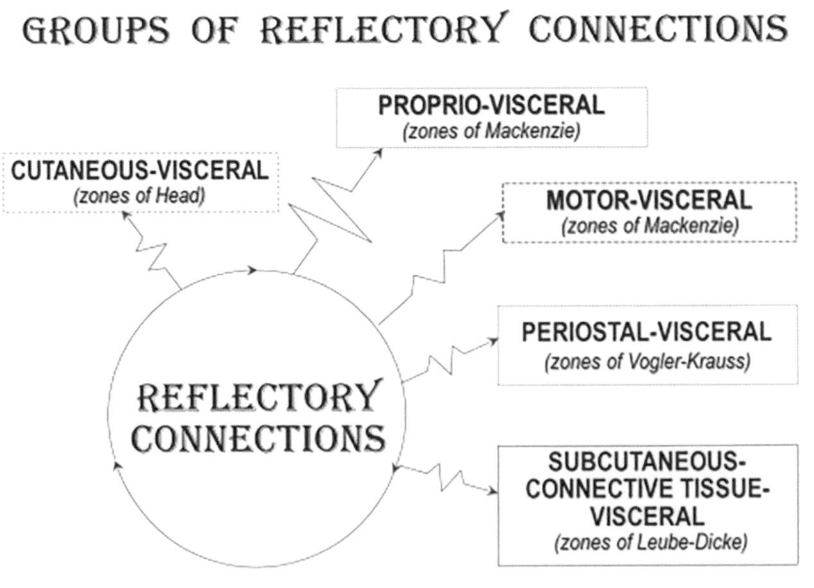

Figure 1.
Groups of reflectory connections.

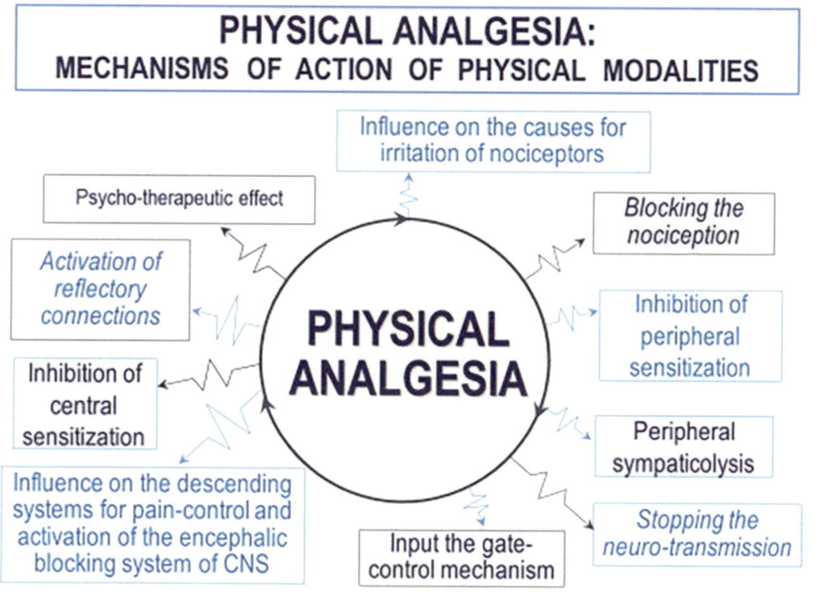

Figure 2.
Mechanisms of physical analgesia.

Mechanism of physical analgesia	Procedures with physical modalities, using this mechanism
By influence on the cause for irritation of pain receptors	Low and medium frequency electric currents, magnetic field, ultrasound, He-Ne laser; massages; manual techniques
By blocking of nociception	Low frequency currents, including transcutaneous electrical nerve stimulation or TENS; lasertherapy
By inhibition of peripheral senzitization	Low and middle frequency currents, TENS; magnetic field; lasertherapy
By peripheral sympaticolysis	Low frequency currents e.g. dyadinamic currents, peloids
By stopping the neural transmission (by C and Aδ delta—fibers) to the body of the first neuron of the general sensibility	Iontophoresis with Novocain in the receptive zone—the region of neuro-terminals
By input of the gate-control mechanism	TENS with frequency 90–130 Hz and interferential currents with high resulting frequency—90-150 Hz
By activation of the reflectory connections	classic manual, connective tissue and periostal massage, post-isometric relaxation and stretching-techniques
By influence on the pain-translation at the level of posterior horn of the spinal medulla—using the root of activation of encephalic blocking system in the central nervous system (increasing the peripheral afferentation) and influence on the descending systems for pain—control	TENS with frequency 2–5 Hz and interferential currents with low resulting frequency 1–5 Hz, acupuncture and laserpuncture; reflectory and periostal massage, zonotherapy, acupressure, su-dgok massage; preformed factors in reflectory zones /palms of hands, plants of feet, paravertebral points; zones of Head, of Mackenzie, of Leube-Dicke, of Vogler-Krauss/
By inhibition of central sensitization	Lasertherapy; peloidotherapy; physiotherapy
By influence on the psychic state of the patient—the drug «doctor» and the drug «procedure».	Regular procedures with physical modalities

Table 2.
Mechanism of physical analgesia and correspondent procedures.

- *By influence on the cause for irritation of pain receptors*—consequence of stimulation of circulation, metabolism and trophy of tissues;
- *By blocking of nociception*;
- *By inhibition of peripheral senzitization*;
- *By peripheral sympaticolysis*;
- *By stopping the neural transmission (by C and Aδ delta—fibers) to the body of the first neuron of the general sensibility*;
- *By input of the gate-control mechanism*;
- *By activation of different reflectory connections*;
- *By influence on the pain-translation at the level of the posterior horn of the spinal medulla—using the root of activation of encephalic blocking system in the central nervous system* (increasing the peripheral afferentation) and *influence on the descending systems for pain—control*;
- *By inhibition of central sensitization*;
- *By influence on the psychic state of the patient*—the drug "doctor" and the drug "procedure".

4. Physical analgesia: systematic mechanisms

Physical modalities influence at different levels: on the cells and the interstitium, especially on the cellular membrane and on mitochondrial membranes; on the neuron and neuroglia; on systematic level; on psychic condition of the patient (psycho-emotional stress of chronic pain).

Low frequency electric currents, Deep oscillation, lasertherapy and active physiotherapy have influence on different mechanisms of cellular alteration, as follows: ischemic, hypoxic, hypo-energetic, oxidative stress.

Some rehabilitation procedures stimulate active hyperemia: electrotherapy, magnetic field, active physiotherapy, hydro- and balneo-therapy, acupuncture.

Other agents reduce passive hyperemia: magnetotherapy, deep oscillation, manual massage, manual lymphatic drainage and lymphopressotherapy, active physiotherapy.

Some procedures influence on the exudative phase of inflammation, reducing exudates: high frequency electric currents, laser, deep oscillation, lymphatic drainage, manual massage, active physiotherapy.

Physical modalities reduce systematic effects of inflammation. Active physiotherapy, manual massage and reflectory techniques reduce toxo-infectious syndrome. Active and passive physiotherapy, lasertherapy and ultra-violet light therapy reduce the asteno-adynamic syndrome. Active physiotherapy and reflectory techniques reduce C-reactive protein, regulate endocrinium, and regulate the balance between sympaticus and parasympathicus.

Active physiotherapeutic procedures reduce hypoxia (hypoxic, circulatory and tissue hypoxia) and stimulate compensatory mechanisms (respiratory, cardio-vascular and tissular).

Physical modalities ameliorate the function of the central and peripheral nervous system. Low frequency electric currents (iontophoresis, functional electrical stimulations) have influence on neuronal dysfunction. Physiotherapy, transcranial electric and magnetic stimulations stimulate the function of neuronal groups, chains and nets. Active physiotherapy and ergotherapy improve the cerebral function, acting on cerebral ischaemia, the brain oedema and the intracranial hypertension.

5. Physical analgesia: pros and contras

Physical analgesia is a cheap treatment, accepted positively by patients. Physical procedures have not significant side effects and contra-indications.

The treatment is not difficult for realization, is relatively cheap.

We can combine different rehabilitation procedures. We can combine physical analgesia with other types of analgesia.

We must admit that actually there is a *lack of sufficient evidence* in the area of physical analgesia.

An interdisciplinary team (of medical doctors — specialists in Neurology, Neurosurgery, Rheumatology, Orthopedics and Traumatology, Physical and Rehabilitation Medicine) programs rehabilitation. For practical realization of the procedures, we need a staff of physiotherapists, occupational therapists, nurses, etc.

6. General algorithm for pain management

Pain management with physical modalities is based on traditions of physical and rehabilitation medicine (PRM). According the definition of the European Union of Medical Specialists—PRM Section [12] this is an independent medical specialty, oriented to the promotion of physical and cognitive functioning, activities, participation and changes in personal factors and environment.

According the World Report on Disability of the World Health Organization and World Bank [39] rehabilitation is a functional treatment, based on a detailed functional assessment. Goals of rehabilitation are functional amelioration and functional recovery [39].

The White Book on Physical and Rehabilitation Medicine [12, 13] formulates the basic objective of PRM: increase of patients' quality of life, especially autonomy in everyday activities [40]. Tasks of PRM are oriented to amelioration of functioning and participation in different types of activities [12, 13, 41–43].

Modern rehabilitation algorithm requires a detailed functional evaluation, based on International Classification of Diseases; International Classification of Functioning, disability and Health (ICF) and on clinical principles [44–46]. In rehabilitation clinical practice, we apply a complex rehabilitation programme, combination of different physical factors, in some cases—with drugs.

We consider that the complex algorithm for pain management must include: systematic drugs (and vitamins); rehabilitation complex, and patient education.

The complex PRM algorithm includes a detailed functional assessment of the patient and a complex rehabilitation programme. Functional evaluation emphasizes on goniometry, manual muscle test, grasp and gait evaluation, autonomy in everyday activities, ICF evaluation, Visual analogue scale for pain /VAS 0-10/, McGill Pain questionnaire) [47]. The rehabilitation program is established by synergic combination of different natural and preformed physical modalities (kinesiotherapy and ergotherapy, cryo and peloido-procedures, electrotherapy and photo-therapy, magnetic field, etc.). This program must include: *one or two pre-formed modalities; one thermo- or kryo-agent; one or two physiotherapeutic procedures* (including analytic exercises, soft tissue techniques, manual therapy, etc.).

At the end of every rehabilitation course, it is obligatory to realize a functional assessment—with the goal to evaluate the efficacy and to prescribe the consecutive rehabilitation procedures.

During our modest clinical experience (of 30 years) we received multiple significant results in patients with conditions of the nervous and motor systems [48–52]. We realized comparative evaluation between the efficacy of pure drug therapy, physical analgesia and combined anti-pain therapy *(drug and physical analgesia)* on different types of pain: spastic pain; rigidity pain; hemiparetic shoulder pain and hemiplegic hand pain; paravertebral (upper & low back) pain; radicular neuropathic pain; diabetic polyneuropathy pain; arthrosis pain; arthritis pain; scoliotic pain; post-traumatic pain; post-operative pain; phantom pain.

7. Pathogenetic base of PRM-programs for pain management

The influence of physical modalities on the interstitium (*milieu intérieur* of Claude Bernard) is the theoretical base for combination of drugs and physical modalities [53, 54].

The synergy between different physical modalities is the logical base for prescription of complex rehabilitation program. According the theory of Ferreira (1983) pain is a consequence of the combination of algesic and hyperalgesic stimulation [54]. Natural physical modalities (physiotherapy, hydrotherapy, ergotherapy) provoke a block of the hyperalgesic stimulation. The algesic stimulation is influenced by pre-formed physical factors (electric currents, magnetic field, light, etc.). The combination of natural and preformed physical modalities can reduce pain, using different paths.

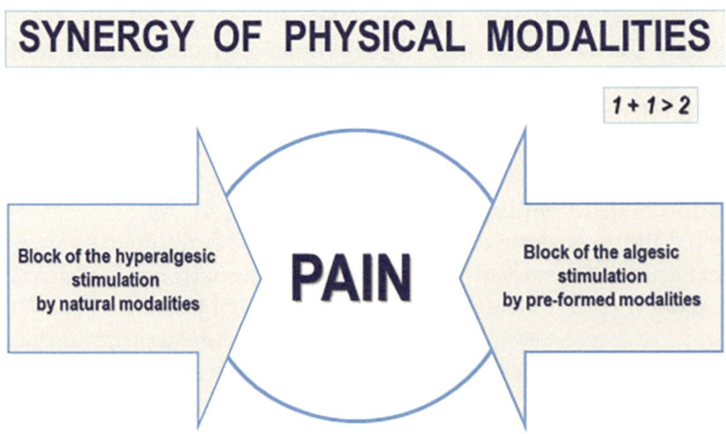

Figure 3.
Synergic combination of physical modalities in pain patients.

The construction of a complex physical and rehabilitation programme is needed, because the mechanism of action of different procedures is diverse (**Figure 3**).

8. Rehabilitation team for pain patients

The obligatory condition for the staff in Pain management is to have competencies in several thematic fields: Pain theories and the correspondent clinical field.

From the point of view of rehabilitation, the objective must be to assure the quality of life and the dignity of these patients. Our problem is the quality of care of pain patients. For us the most important is to guarantee the quality of life of pain patient.

The multi-disciplinary multi-professional team for pain patients must include:

- Medical doctors: specialists in Pain medicine, Neurology, Neurosurgery, Oncology (Neuro-Oncology), Anesthesiology, Radiology (Neuroradiology), Orthopedics and Traumatology; Physical and Rehabilitation Medicine;

- Medical and para-medical staff: Physiotherapist, Ergotherapist (occupational therapist), Nurse, Dietitian, Psychologist, Sociologist, etc.

9. Functional assessment of pain patients

Functional assessment in PRM-practice is based on ICF (**Figure 4**).

The holistic approach to the patient must be obligatory—the complex evaluation must include:

- *Cognitive capacities* (orientation, memory, attention, compliance during rehabilitation, conscience of necessity of preventive measures due to the principal disease);

- *Pain* (localization, type, intensity /verbal or visual analogue scale/; activities increasing pain);

- *Range of motion* (active and passive);

- *Muscle force or muscle weakness*, motor deficiency;

- *Coordination* (static, locomotor or dynamic ataxia);

- *Mobility* (necessity of technical aids, gadgets; instruments, etc.);

- *Endurance* (capacity to support extreme changes, necessity of pauses during investigations and functional activity);

- *Independence in activities of daily living* (bathing, dressing, eating, hygiene, necessity of assistance in self-care).

We evaluate some problems of the pain patient: *Reduced endurance and supportability to physical activity, fatigue; Motor weakness; Coordination problems* (posture, locomotion,

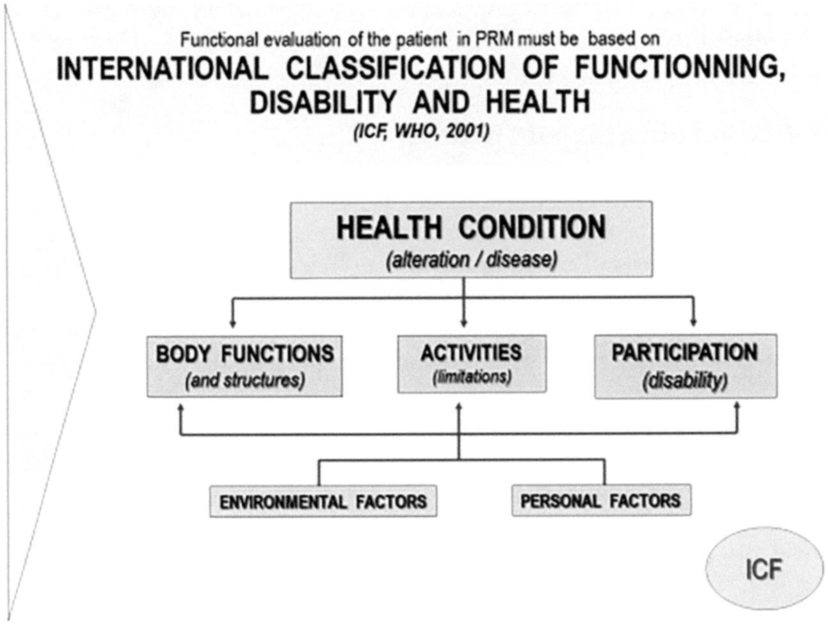

Figure 4.
ICF.

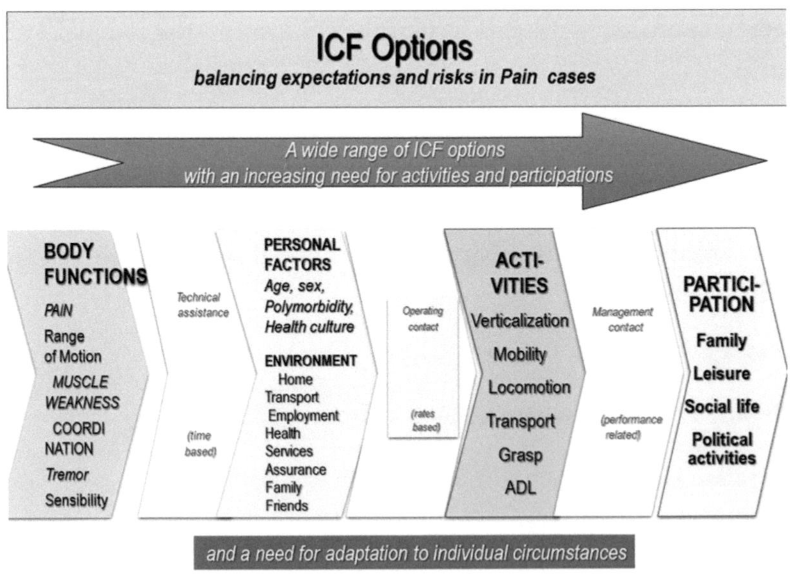

Figure 5.
Assessment of pain patient, based on ICF.

grasping); *Pain; Necessity of preventive measures; Necessity of technical aids; Necessity of assistance; Difficulties in activities of daily living; Reduced performance and Reduced functional mobility.*

The final complex evaluation, based on ICF, have to include (**Figure 5**).

- *Body functions* (pain, range of motion, motor weakness, dyscoordination syndromes—ataxia);
- *Activities* (verticalization, mobility, standing up, walking, transport, grasping, activities of daily living—ADL);
- *Participation* (family life, leisure, social life, participation in political activities);
- *Environmental factors* (environment at home & at work, family & friends, health insurance, health assurance, social contacts);
- *Personal factors* (health culture, polimorbidity, age, sex).

10. Algorithms of pain management in post-operative cases

In every case, including post-operative cases, we apply the same algorithm: detailed functional assessment and complex rehabilitation. This complex rehabilitation principle comprises a synergic combination of different physical modalities and techniques, accentuating on physiotherapy, ergotherapy, functional electrical stimulations and pain management with preformed modalities (**Figure 6**).

We emphasize on strictly analgesic procedures, as follows:

- *From the group of preformed modalities*: dyadinamic electric currents, transcutaneous electroneurostimulation (TENS), Trabert current, interferential currents, magnetic field, LASER, Deep Oscillation, Shock-Wave therapy;

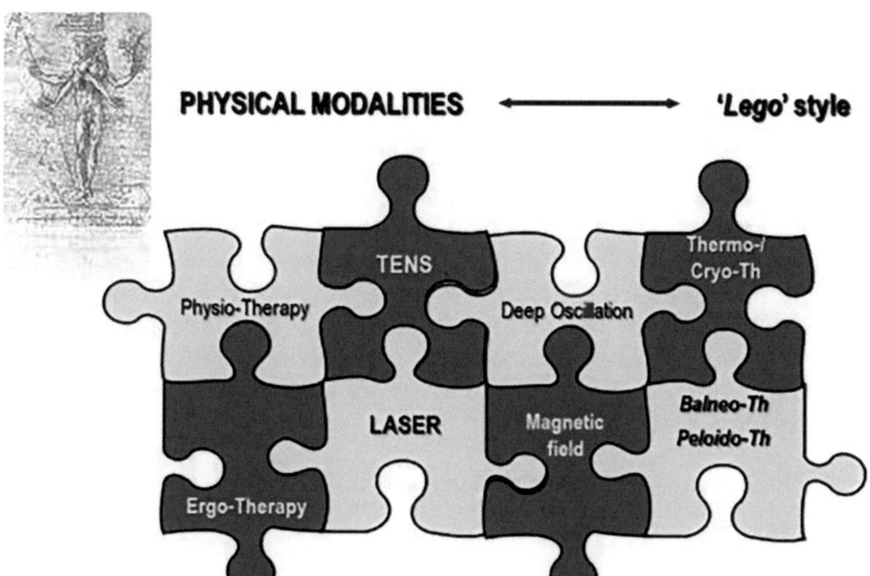

Figure 6.
Rehabilitation puzzle in post-operative cases.

- *From the group of natural physical modalities*: soft tissue techniques (post-isometric relaxation, relaxing massage), manual therapy, extension therapies, balneophysiotherapy, peloidotherapy;

- *From the group of reflectory methods*: acupuncture, low frequency electric currents in reflectory points.

The choice of the concrete physical factor and of the respective therapeutic method depends on the type of pain and of the principal disease or condition [55–59], as follows:

- In nociceptive pain—we apply low frequency electric current (galvanic current, Lidocaine-iontophoresis, dyadinamic current, especially diphase fixe—DF); position therapy, infiltration therapy;

- In neuropathic pain—we prefer transcutaneous electroneurostimulation (TENS), Interferential currents, Deep Oscillation; balneotherapy, peloidotherapy;

- Rheumatic pain in degenerative articular diseases: magnetic field, middle frequency electric currents; laser-therapy, Deep Oscillation; isometric exercises; infiltration therapy (in the joint or around it);

- Rheumatic pain in inflammatory joint diseases: in the acute stage—low and middle frequency electric currents, magnetic field, cryotherapy, analytic isometric exercises; in the chronic stage—interferential currents, magnetic field, Deep Oscillation, laser; balneotherapy, peloidotherapy, passive physiotherapy;

- In post-traumatic conditions: cryotherapy, position therapy, active exercises (accentuating on isometric exercises), magnetotherapy, interferential currents;

- In cases with myofascial pain—middle-frequency electric currents, deep oscillation, stretching of the respective fascia; analytic exercises—against gravity and against resistance; underwater exercises, underwater douche massage;

- In ligamentar pain—shock wave therapy, TENS, cryotherapy, underwater exercises;

- In spondylogenic pain (vertebrogenic and discogenic)—low-frequency electric currents, post-isometric relaxation (PIR), stretching, extension therapy (extension vertebrotherapy), manual therapy (tractions, mobilizations, manipulations), in chronic stage—ultrasound (or phonophoresis with a non-steroidal anti-inflammatory gel), LASER (lasertherapy, laserpuncture, laseracupuncture), exercises for muscular belt, paravertebral infiltrations;

- In oncologic pain—infiltration therapy, active physiotherapy.

During the preparation of the rehabilitation complex, we must combine synergically procedures with three or more mechanisms of physical analgesia.

In some cases, we must combine physical analgesia and medications.

Patient's education is obligatory in cases with chronic pain, especially after surgical intervention.

In the scientific literature, exist some investigations, proving the effectiveness of physical analgesia (with different level of evidence) after surgical interventions. Some of the used combinations are:

- In patients after orthopedic surgery (hip, knee or shoulder arthroplasty; metallic osteosynthesis of long bones of extremities)—mechanotherapy, active exercises for limbs muscles, cryotherapy, interferential currents, Deep Oscillation, functional electrical stimulations, telerehabilitation [10, 24, 25, 30, 31, 33–35, 49, 51, 52];

- In patients after mini-invasive operation of ruptured ligaments—TENS, Interferential currents, Deep Oscillation, magnetic field, laser, analytic exercises, mechanotherapy [23, 49];

- In patients after neurosurgical intervention for brain tumors—mechanotherapy, active exercises, proprioceptive neuromuscular stimulation, balance and gait training [49];

- In patients after operation of discal hernia—TENS, dyadinamic currents, interferential currents, Deep Oscillation; Magnetic field, lasertherapy; analytic exercises, position therapy, relaxing massage, gait training [10, 17, 22, 31, 33, 49, 50];

- In patients after limb amputation with stump pain and phantom pain—Deep Oscillation, Lasertherapy, analytic exercises [26, 48];

- In patients after abdominal operations: active exercises, electrical stimulations for stimulation of the peristaltic [26].

11. Conclusion

Pain management is an important part of rehabilitation algorithms in clinical practice. PRM-programmes of care is obligatory in pain cases, especially in post-operative patients.

We could recommend our complex pain management program.

The on-time start of rehabilitation procedures in pain management (especially after surgical intervention) has a lot of beneficial consequences: improvement of patient condition and prevention of complications; increase of muscle force and range of motion; regularization of static and balance; normalization of humero-scapular and pelvi-femoral rhythm; functional recovery of the grasp and gait, amelioration of autonomy of patients and of quality of life; acceleration of resocialization and participation in functional activities, positive economic effect.

Conflict of interest

The authors declare no conflicts of interest.

Author details

Ivet B. Koleva[1,2,3]*, Borislav R. Yoshinov[4], Teodora A. Asenova[4] and Radoslav R. Yoshinov[5]

1 Medical University of Sofia, Bulgaria

2 Specialized Hospital for Long-Term Care and Rehabilitation "Serdika" with Medical Center for Robotic Neurorehabilitation "ReGo"- Sofia, Bulgaria

3 Physical Medicine Department, National Heart Hospital, Sofia, Bulgaria

4 Medical Faculty of Sofia University, Bulgaria

5 University for Library Studies and Information Technologies, Sofia, Bulgaria

*Address all correspondence to: dr.yvette.5@gmail.com

References

[1] International Association for the Study of Pain. Pain – Definition. 2008. Available from: www.iasp-pain.org

[2] Koleva I, Yoshinov R, Yoshinov B. Physical analgesia. Monograph. Saint-Denis, France, "Connaissances et savoirs". Science. 2018;**2018**:146

[3] Descartes R. L'homme de René Descartes. Paris: Charles Angot; 1664

[4] Noordenbos W. Pain: Problems Pertaining to the Transmission of Nerve Impulses, Which Give Rise to Pain. Amsterdam: Elsevier; 1959

[5] Melzack R, Wall PD. Pain mechanisms: A new theory. Science. 1965;**150**:971-979

[6] Wall P. The gait control theory of pain mechanisms. A re-examination and re-statement. Brain. 1978;**101**(1):1-18

[7] Melzack R. From the gate to the neuromatrix. Pain. 1999;**Suppl 6**: S121-S126

[8] Calcutt NA, Dunn JS. Pain: Nociceptive and neuropathic mechanisms. Anesthesiology Clinics of North America. 1997;**15**:429-444

[9] Merskey H, Bogduk N, editors. Classification of Chronic Pain – Descriptions of Chronic Pain Syndromes and Definition of Pain Terms. Seattle: IASP press; 1994

[10] Koleva I. Physical Analgesia and Deep Oscillation. Sofia: SIMEL; 2015

[11] Declaration of Montreal. Available from: www.iasp-pain.org

[12] Gutenbrunner C, Ward AB, Chamberlain MA. Editors. White book on Physical and rehabilitation medicine in Europe. Journal of Rehabilitation Medicine. 2007;**45**(1):s1-s48. Available from: www.medicaljournals.se/jrm

[13] European Physical and Rehabilitation Medicine Bodies Alliance. White Book on Physical and Rehabilitation Medicine in Europe. Third edition. European Journal of Physical and Rehabilitation Medicine. 2018;**54**(2):1-204

[14] Koleva I, Yoshinov B, Yoshinov RR. Perspectives in pain management: Physical analgesia. Medical Journal of Clinical Trials Case Studies. 2018;**2**(1):1-3

[15] Koleva I. Chronic pain and physical analgesia: The impact of physical modalities to reduce pain. Journal of Biomedical and Clinical Research. 2008;**1**(1):12-17

[16] Reynes C. Neuropathie diabetique peripherique: Reponses vasomotrices. France: d'Avignon Universite. Avignon; 2021

[17] Radeva St, Zaralieva A, Tonev D. Predetermined physical factors and alternative factors in the treatment of chronic pain in discogenic lumbosacral radiculitis. Reumatologia. 2022;**60**(2):110-115

[18] Sluka K, Walsh D. Transcutaneous electrical nerve stimulation: basic science mechanisms and clinical effectiveness. Journal of Pain. 2003;**4**(3):109-121

[19] Walsh DM, Foster NE, Baxter GD. Trancutaneous electrical nerve stimulation. Relevance of stimulation parameters to neurophysiological and hypoalgesic effects. American Journal of Physical Medicine and Rehabilitation. 1995;**74**(3):199-206

[20] Johnson M. The clinical effectiveness of TENS in pain management. Critical Reviews in Physical and Rehabilitation Medicine. 2000;**12**(2):131-149

[21] Koleva I, Iochinov RD, Zl S, et al. Transcutaneous electroneurostimulation and fangotherapy in diabetic polyneuropathy patients. In: Abstracts Book of the Third World Congress in Neurological Rehabilitation. Venice, Italy; 2002. p. 497

[22] Koleva I. Interdisciplinary approach towards analgesia in low back pain and lumbo-sacral radiculopathy: Impact of paravertebral infiltrations, laser therapy and deep oscillation (a comparative study of five rehabilitation complexes). International Journal of Anesthesiology & Pain Medicine. 2019;**5**:21-22. DOI: 10.21767/2471-982X-C1-004

[23] Koleva I, Yoshinov B, Bayraktarova A, Yoshinov RR. Impact of magnetic field and deep oscillation in the complex rehabilitation after arthroscopic reconstruction of the anterior cruciate ligament (a comparative study). Journal of Medical and Clinical Studies. 2020;**3**(1):130. www.pubtexto.com

[24] Mratskova G. Use of deep oscillation therapy in rehabilitation program for patient after distal radius fracture with a complex regional pain syndrome: A case report. Trakia Journal of Sciences. 2020;**18**(Suppl.1):187-193

[25] Koleva I, Yoshinov B, Yoshinov R, Asenova T. Physical analgesia and functional recovery in hip and knee osteoarthritis: Rehabilitation algorithms. Archives of Rheumatology and Arthritis Research. 2022;**2**(3):1-7. DOI: 10.33552/ARAR.2022.02.000539

[26] Koleva I. Repetitorium physiotherapeuticum (basic principles of the modern physical and rehabilitation medicine). In: Book for English Speaking Students. Sofia: Publishing house "SIMEL"; 2008

[27] Lewit K. Postisometric relaxation in combination with other methods of muscular facilitation and inhibition. Man and Medicine. 1986;**2**:101-104

[28] Lewit K. Manipulative Therapy in the Rehabilitation of the Locomotor System. Second ed. London: Butterworth; 1991. pp. 30-32

[29] Maigne R. Diagnostic et traitement des douleurs communes d'origine rachidienne. Paris: Expansion Scientifique Française; 1989 p.301-8, 395-404

[30] Maraver F, Roques CF, Karagulle MZ, Inokuma S, Surdu O, et al. Analisis bibliometrico de los WC ISMH (2010-2019). Biological Sociology Esp Hidrological Medicine. 2021;**36**(1):9-26

[31] Koleva I, Krastev N, Yoshinov R. Impact of balneotherapy and peloidotherapy in neurorehabilitation algorithm of patients with low back pain and lumbo-sacral radiculopathy – A comparative study. Balnea. 2015;**10**:87-88 Serie de Monografías; ISBN: 978-84-606-9368-0

[32] Rosino J, Legido-Soto JL, Mourelle-Mosqueira ML, Gomez-Perez CP, Navarro-Garcia JR. La Peloterapia: historia, caracteristicas y propiedades. Agua y Territorio. 2020;**17**:111-130

[33] Koleva I, Yoshinov R, Marinov M, Hadjijanev A. Efficacy of hydro-, balneo- and peloidotherapy in the pain management and quality of life of patients with socially-important diseases and conditions of the locomotory and nervous system: Bulgarian experience. Balnea. 2015;**10**:273-274 Serie de Monografías; ISBN: 978-84-606-9368-0

[34] Che J-Y, Da-Yong L. Acupuncture for bone disease treatments. EC Orthopaedics. 2020;**12**(1):15-16

[35] Xie SH, Wang Q, Wang LQ, Wang L, Song KP, He CQ. Effect of internet-based rehabilitation programs on improvement of pain and physical function in patients with knee osteoarthritis: Systematic review and meta-analysis of randomized controlled trials. Journal of Medical Internet Research. 2021;**23**(1):1-13 e215442

[36] Tsang MP, Man GCW, Xin H, Chong YC, Ong MTY, et al. The effectiveness of telerehabilitation in patients after total knee replacement: A systematic review and meta-analysis of randomized controlled trials. Journal of Telemedicine and Telecare. 2022:1-14 SAGE, DOI: 10.1177/1357633X221097469

[37] Gacheva J. Diagnostics and Therapy with Low Frequency Currents. Sofia: Medizina & Fizkultura; 1980. p. 204

[38] Terenius L. Profiles of CSF neuropeptides in chronic pain of different nature. In: Sicuteri F, Terenius L, Vecchiet L, Maggi C, editors. Advances of Pain Research and Therapy. 1992. pp. 93-100

[39] World Health Organization and the World Bank. World Report on Disability. Geneva: WHO Press; 2011

[40] American Academy of Physical Medicine and Rehabilitation Task Force on Medical Inpatient Rehabilitation Criteria (JL Melvin Chair). Standards for Assessing Medical Appropriateness Criteria for Admitting Patients to Rehabilitation Hospitals or Units. 2006. Available at: http://www.aapmr.org / hpl/legislation/ mirc.htm [Accessed: March 13, 2008]

[41] Haig AJ. Practice of physical medicine and rehabilitation on both sides of the Atlantic: Differences and the factors that drive them. European Journal of Physical and Rehabilitation Medicine. 2008;**44**(2):111-115

[42] DeLisa JA. Physical Medicine and Rehabilitation – Principles and Practice. Fourth ed. Philadelphia: Lippincott, Williams & Wilkins; 2005

[43] Melvin JL. Physical and rehabilitation medicine: Comments related to the white book on physical and rehabilitation medicine in Europe. European Journal of Physical and Rehabilitation Medicine. 2008;**44**(2):117-119

[44] World Health Organization. The ICD-10 Classification of Mental and Behavioral Disorders: Clinical Descriptors and Diagnostic Guidelines. 10th ed. Geneva: WHO; 1992

[45] World Health Organization. International Classification of Functioning, Disability and Health (ICF). Geneva: WHO; 2001

[46] Stucki G, Ewert T, Cieza A. Value and application of the ICF in rehabilitation medicine. Disability and Rehabilitation. 2002;**24**:932-938

[47] Melzack R. The short-form McGill questionnaire. Pain. 1987;**30**:191-197

[48] Koleva I, Ioshinov B, Yoshinov RD. Potential of physical analgesia in the complex rehabilitation of patients with stump pain and phantom pain after lower limb amputation (a double-blind randomised controlled trial of efficacy of Deep Oscillation, Laser therapy and Paravertebral infiltrations). In: Book Publisher International: Current Trends in Medicine and Medical Research. Vol.3, Chapter 9; pp. 74-94. Print ISBN: 978-93-89246-02-5, eBook ISBN: 978-93-89246-46-9

[49] Koleva IB, Avramescu ET. Grasp and Gait Rehabilitation (Bases). Monograph. Sofia: Simel Press; 2017. p. 394

[50] Koleva I, Marinov MB. Impact of deep oscillation in the complex rehabilitation algorithm for patients after spinal neurosurgery. Eurasian Union of Scientists (EUS). 2015;**21**(12):78-82 ISSN 2411-6467.

[51] Koleva I, Avramescu E, Kamal D, Kamal C, Traistaru MR. Rehabilitation guidelines of operational standard procedures in rehabilitation after lower limb orthopedic surgery. In: Education and New Developments. Lisbon: Mafalda Carmo; 2017. pp. 594-598

[52] Koleva I, Yoshinov B, Papathanassiou J, Hadjiyanev A. Necessity of inclusion of muscular belt training exercises in the complex rehabilitation programme of osteoarthritic patients after Total hip replacement (A case report). Journal of Medical and Clinical Studies. 2020;**3**(1):133

[53] Burnstock G. A unifying purinergic hypothesis for the initiation of pain. Lancet. 1996;**347**:1604-1605

[54] Ferreira SH. Prostaglandins: Peripheral and central analgesia. In: Bonicca JJ et al., editors. Advances in Pain Research and Therapy. Vol. 5. New York: Raven Press; 1983. pp. 627-634

[55] Koleva I, Yoshinov B, Gerenova G, Yoshinov RR. Geriatric rehabilitation: program of care after orthopedic surgery for proximal femoral fractures. Medcrave; MOJ Gerontology & Geriatrics. 2020;**5**:133-140. DOI: 10.15406/ mojgg.2020.05.00245. eISSN: 2574-8130

[56] Hansjurgens A, May HU. Grundlagen der Elektrotherapie. Karlsruhe: Nemectron GmbH; 2003

[57] Hayes KW. Manual for Physical Agents. New Jersey: Prentice Hall Health; 2003. p. 209

[58] Nalty T, Sabbahi M. Nalty T, editor. Electrotherapy Clinical Procedures Manual. New York: McGraw – Hill; 2001. p. 299

[59] Fulop AM, Dhimmer S, Deluca JR, Johanson DD, Lenz RV, Patel KB, et al. A meta-analysis of the efficacy of laser phototherapy on pain relief. The Clinical Journal of Pain. 2010;**26**:729-736